Hidden Attractions of Administration

This book argues that the expansion of administrative activities in today's working life is driven not only by pressure from above, but also from below. The authors examine the inner dynamics of people-processing organizations—those formally working for clients, patients, or students—to uncover the hidden attractions of doing administrative work, despite all the complaints and laments about "too many meetings" or "too much paperwork." There is something appealing to those compelled to participate in today's constantly multiplying and expanding administration that defies popular framings of it as merely pressure from above. *Hidden Attractions of Administration* shows in detail the emotional attractiveness, moral conflicts, and almost magical features that administrative tasks often entail in today's organizations, supported by ethnographic studies consisting of over 200 qualitative interviews and participant observations from ten organizational settings and contexts across Sweden. The authors also question and complement explanations in administration-related research that have previously been taken for granted, arguing that it is a simplification to attribute all aspects of the change to New Public Management and instead taking into account what the classic sociologist Georg Simmel called an *Eigendynamik*: a self-reinforcing tendency that, under certain circumstances, needs only a nudge in an administrative direction to get going. By applying ethnography to issues of bureaucratization and meeting cultures and by drawing on findings in emotional sociology and social anthropology, this volume contributes to both the sociology of work and the study of human service organizations and will appeal to scholars and students working across both areas.

Malin Åkerström is a professor of sociology in the Department of Sociology, Lund University, Sweden.

Katarina Jacobsson is a professor of social work in the School of Social Work, Lund University, Sweden.

Erika Andersson Cederholm is an associate professor in the Department of Service Management and Service Studies, Lund University, Sweden.

David Wästerfors is a professor of sociology in the Department of Sociology, Lund University, Sweden.

Routledge Studies in the Sociology of Work, Professions, and Organizations

This series presents the latest sociological and social scientific research on professions, work and organizations, welcoming studies of careers, professional motivations, organizational change, entrepreneurship, workplace issues, working lives and identities, labor relations, and the transformation of work in a changing economy.

Titles in this series:

Identity, Motivation, and Memory
The Role of History in the British and German Forces
Sarah Katharina Kayss

Working Lives and in-House Outsourcing
Chewed-Up by Two Masters
Jacqueline M. Zalewski

The Construction Precariat
Dependence, Domination, and Labor in Dhaka
Selim Reza

Hidden Attractions of Administration
The Peculiar Appeal of Meetings and Documents
Malin Åkerström, Katarina Jacobsson, Erika Andersson Cederholm, and David Wästerfors

For more information about this series, please visit: https://www.routledge.com/Routledge-Studies-in-the-Sociology-of-Work-Professions-and-Organisations/book-series/RSSWPO

Hidden Attractions of Administration

The Peculiar Appeal of Meetings and Documents

**Malin Åkerström,
Katarina Jacobsson,
Erika Andersson Cederholm,
and David Wästerfors**

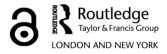

Routledge
Taylor & Francis Group

LONDON AND NEW YORK

First published 2021
by Routledge
2 Park Square, Milton Park, Abingdon, Oxon OX14 4RN

and by Routledge
605 Third Avenue, New York, NY 10158

Routledge is an imprint of the Taylor & Francis Group, an informa business

© 2021 Malin Åkerström, Katarina Jacobsson, Erika Andersson Cederholm, and David Wästerfors

The right of Malin Åkerström, Katarina Jacobsson, Erika Andersson Cederholm, and David Wästerfors to be identified as authors of this work has been asserted by them in accordance with sections 77 and 78 of the Copyright, Designs and Patents Act 1988.

British Library Cataloguing-in-Publication Data
A catalogue record for this book is available from the British Library

Library of Congress Cataloging-in-Publication Data
A catalog record has been requested for this book

ISBN: 978-0-367-62227-5 (hbk)
ISBN: 978-0-367-62226-8 (pbk)
ISBN: 978-1-003-10843-6 (ebk)

DOI: 10.4324/9781003108436

Typeset in Garamond
by MPS Limited, Dehradun

Contents

Acknowledgments

We want to thank the following persons for valuable comments, suggestions, and inspiration during our work with this book: Goran Basic, Lisa Carlstedt, Lisa Flower, Teres Hjärpe, Maggie Kusenbach, Christina McKnight, Elizabeth Martinell Barfoed, Susie Scott, Helen Schwartzman, Ann-Mari Sellerberg, Joakim Thelander, and Sophia Yakhlef. We also want to thank the very encouraging reviewer of a sample of this manuscript, as well as the editor at SF Edit who made an exceptionally careful reading of our text. The Swedish Research Council has financed the project that made this book possible (project nr. 2016-02901).

Preface

It might seem that this is a critical book about the administration society and its contemporary expansion, and in a way that is right. It is easy to get appalled—there is something quite provocative in people's engagement in paperwork and meetings at the expense of "proper" work, especially when there is a client somewhere in the organization, waiting for some attention.

Still we have turned this and other emotions into a topic rather than a motive for our writing (since field members may very well feel the same) and instead subsumed our efforts to something else: wonder. The book is written out of our amazement of the expanding administration. These relentless efforts to document more and more, and to call for more and more meetings, how do people go about making them accountable and attractive?

In *Osebol*, a prize-winning collection of poems written by Marit Kapla (2019) based on interviews with villagers, a whole community is portrayed, situated in Värmland, a province in West-central Sweden. They talk about their life, their background, their mundane feelings, and their surroundings. It is surprising—and yet logical—that an increased demand to administer have found its way also to this place and text, including the sighing and wonder.

In one poem, one of the narrators touches upon night shifts in a nursing home, which is her job. "But there is a lot of administrative stuff," she says, "having become so central" (our translation from Swedish). "One should write / and note things in the computer" instead of spending time with the clients.

> It would be very nice
> if one could hear sometime
> that put this aside
> and sit down together with the elderly

The narrator Mona goes on and says that they once were required to write up all details regarding what they did to assist the elderly in each room. It resulted in a sizeable pile of information, considering that they took care of 23 people, and visited their rooms several times. In an ironic tone, she notes:

The only thing we would not write up
was which foot
we entered the room with

What an energy it takes, the narrator concludes, "instead of putting the energy/on the human being."

Once we had five A4 papers
on both sides
that we had written
about one person
during one night

Who will ever read and remember, Mona asks herself in the poem, what is written on those papers?

So, the topic of this book is not exclusive for the offices and webpages of urban workplaces, with their neat conference rooms and fancy coffee machines. It stretches out to almost every corner and margin of society, even to a remote little village in mid-Sweden's countryside.

Malin Åkerström
Katarina Jacobsson
Erika Andersson Cederholm
David Wästerfors
Lund, Sweden, October 2020

1 Eigendynamik

> "Wouldn't it help to have a checklist, in these situations?" Lisa, a social worker, asks. She finds it hard to know exactly what to say to parents when they are to be told that they have been reported for maltreatment of their children. "When I came here [to this social services unit] I discovered there was nothing" – no formal guidelines, no checklist. /---/ In her talk with her colleagues during this working group meeting, Lisa argues that they should write up what they should say at meetings with the families, so that these encounters are ordered from now on. Otherwise "it's unclear what we do." "What are we really doing?" (fieldnotes from the social services)

What are we really doing? Shouldn't we have a checklist? Today there is a fascination with *turning the social world to administration*: pinpointing all activities, defining them, ordering them, arranging meetings about them, producing texts and tables related to them (and then more texts and tables on these texts and tables), and putting it all into digital systems.

A meeting that fails to end in a request for a document of some sort or the production of a document is hardly seen as successful. Documents are counted as tangible results and expected to be circulated digitally to structure all upcoming meetings. There is a chain of events, especially in today's people-processing organizations, that reproduces and strengthens *the administration society*. "There was nothing," Lisa says in the above-quoted fieldnote, implying that "no documentation" equals "nothing," that the absence of administrative order is the same as a social void. Oral or wordless actions and conventions—undocumented routines or pragmatic ways of working that have not been put into schedules, squares, charts, and legitimized discourses—are downplayed or dismissed in favor of textualized and bureaucratically ordered ones.

No checklist? Won't do. Without written systems with codified activities, there is no clarity, and without meetings, "nothing" is happening during a workday. Without figures and schedules, acronyms and webpages, boxes and arrows, there is no distinct idea of an organization. Without administrative accounts of an action, the action as such becomes almost unreal—as if it

DOI: 10.4324/9781003108436-1

never happened. In fact, documents are the only permanent signs that, for example, social work (as in this case) has taken place or will do so. The documents come into existence before or long after any eventual concrete activity and physical interaction have occurred: they are tangible, respected, formal, and proper. Documentation—along with the meetings producing it—provides the opportunity to demonstrate a systematic, regular, and professional approach (Prior 2003).

This book is about the appeal of these administrative accounts. It deals with the pulls and powers of today's surprisingly expanding administration, but we do not address this tension in terms of conventional organizational sociology. Instead, our approach is more in line with Goffman's dramaturgical analysis of organizations and Simmel's analyses of interaction. It is an ethnographic investigation of "doing administration."

Rather than trying to explain the top-down dynamics of this development (depicted by concepts like the *Audit Society* or *New Public Management*), this book expounds on something relatively neglected: the *inner* dynamics, the *everyday attractions and contingencies* that keep people's appetite for administration alive. We try to analyze the interactive processes that sharpen and boost employees' administrative ambitions in today's society.

The book's inspiration is the classic sociologist Georg Simmel's term *Eigendynamik*, i.e., social processes of interaction that create their own momentum, for which Simmel (1978:119) used the metaphor of the circle. We want to investigate an *Eigendynamik* of administration, where it spins around itself in a self-preserving and self-strengthening way. We argue that when that spin is generated in settings involving strong ideas of rationality and democratizing ideas of "everybody's involvement"—at times creating opposing social forces—it tends to become an expanding spiral.

In addition to discussing expanding administrative spirals, we seek to show how a variety of these spirals work and what forms their everyday attractions. We base our analyses on ethnographic studies of several people-processing organizations in Sweden—in psychiatric care, health care, the social services, youth care, and the border police (for more details, see appendix). We also draw on interviews and fieldnotes as well as personal experiences from academia and our own roles, as those experiences are not exempted from the tendencies we study.

We try to show what or who is left behind or sidestepped. In the above-quoted fieldnote, "parents"—the clients—are mentioned ("to know exactly what to say to the parents …"), but they are not placed at the center. The center is reserved for the checklist, or rather its disturbing and conspicuous absence, along with the comfort and relief that would arise if only somebody could formulate it. If only there were a checklist, goes the implied argument, meetings with families would become correct, exact, good, and proper because staff would finally know exactly what to say and do, and things would be ordered. But what's next?

The spiral expands. The working group meeting we observed could very well be used to discuss this new checklist and specify it, and further meetings could be based on it. There may even be courses developed to train staff on how to use the new checklist properly and instructions that explain its rationale in detail. And these courses must be arranged and coordinated through a series of new meetings, properly documented, evaluated, and accounted for. All checklists at all departments could be reviewed regularly and coordinated by a committee with its own meetings and protocols, as well as a digital system designed for this purpose.

This scenario is not mere invention. In our data, we have seen such sequences unfold again and again. When the administration society expands, the very point of people-processing organizations—or, at least, their formal points—weakens or dissolves. This fade does not happen dramatically or explicitly but subtly, step by step, in an almost unstoppable and self-reinforcing manner. Instead of helping out clients, staff carefully and firmly build up time- and energy-consuming palaces with few if any rooms reserved for concrete clients and their concrete lives. The structure they create is a palace of administration.

A glimpse into everyday dynamics

We walk through the corridors of a big and modern multi-storage housing complex, eventually coming to a quite small conference room with ten chairs around an oval table. Here in the managing section of a public psychiatry practice, a meeting is about to take place. Six unit managers arrive, greeting each other and the chairman, Paul, a district manager. They chat a little bit and start arranging their meeting props: papers, calendars, binders, and laptops. "I usually write my memos directly on the computer," Paul says to our fieldworker Joakim, "so that I don't have to do it afterwards."

The meeting is about psychiatric care. The managers are supposed to exchange information and experiences from their respective patient-treating units once every second week. This meeting starts with Paul's turning it over to a new unit manager, who talks about the tough situation at her ward right now, where they have a heavy workload. Another manager talks about a similar situation at her ward, with staff members quitting all the time. "All right," Paul says after a while, "it's a tough time now." He starts talking about the need to recruit a new secretary, and the others agree. They talk about other ongoing recruitments (among them, an occupational therapist) and their work situation again. They talk about young patients in care who have used narcotics and developed psychiatric problems as a result. Eventually, all participants have reported their situation in their respective unit—they all refer to a heavy workload—and Paul starts talking about the meeting's other issues.

Paul reminds the participants of the "working groups" they had established previously. These groups had meetings on their own to "work actively" with things that concerned them, things that needed to be discussed more "deeply." Paul addresses the assembly as a whole: Wouldn't it be wise to start these working groups again, with a new series of meetings? His suggestion is initially met with some resistance:

> Beth responds immediately: "We do have quite a lot of other things to take care of, I think [instead of meeting in groups]." Others nod and say "uhum." "Well, that's a fact," says Nick, "but if I could say something now ...." "You're talking all the time," says Anne and smiles. "Yes, I hear your voice," Hilma adds. Nick also smiles but goes on: "I think it would be a good idea anyway to have a working group about what we talked about before, namely patients who both abuse drugs and have a psychosis." The others nod, and they all talk about this for a while. Also, Beth says something about such a working group possibly being "sensible." Paul takes a note on his laptop and rounds off the discussions by saying that he has noted the interest and will get back to this.

The meeting then revolves around other things: the documentation of patients taking more than three prescription drugs, whether a physician should be present at their meetings, vacation distribution during an upcoming holiday, and new latch bolts for the patient rooms in the buildings.

Paul's suggestion of renewed working groups is not a blunt or drastic bureaucratization. Rather, it is subtle. It is seemingly trivial in relation to other issues taken up and is just a detail compared to larger problems and more urgent tasks in the workplace, and it is introduced in a delicate and nice way. Paul does not demand new working groups or insist on having any particular manager as a member. He just suggests it, and he refers to the fact that working groups did exist before. Another participant, Nick, helps to anchor Paul's suggestion in a topic that obviously engages his colleagues: patients taking drugs and having psychosis. The clear implication is that the working groups should deal with such things.

Indeed, nothing in our data indicates a hidden agenda here, for instance in terms of Paul's trying to manipulate the managers into accepting working groups even though they do not like them. Our point is different—and sociological. There is an administrative *Eigendynamik* set in motion when Paul articulates his suggestion, and when Beth's spontaneous objection ("We do have quite a lot of other things to take care of") is overruled, there is a spiraling sequence of events that seems hard to stop, despite the initial hesitancy.

When our fieldworker reports from another meeting six weeks after the one described here, with the same participants, Paul's first point on his agenda is the appointment of a working group. Now, the working group unquestionably comes into existence. It will consist of staff within the psychiatry unit as well as the local municipality, and its purpose will be to improve "cooperation." The group will produce a document describing how this cooperation will function, stated "as clearly as possible," as a manager puts it during this meeting. What does this mean?

This means that another administrative forum is created within this organization, with its own series of meetings and associated texts. Another schedule for meetings is emerging, with a plethora of emails, agendas, and protocols. Managers—this time also from the municipality—are drawn into another chain of administrative activities, with merely abstract and very remote significance for patients or the workload in the clinics. The participants still have "quite a lot of other things to take care of," to quote Beth from the first meeting, but they will nonetheless spend time in new meetings and pinpoint new things in new texts that will circulate digitally and require more reading.

The pull and power of the administration society are activated, and implicit ideals of rationality and participation nurture the process. Why not a working group? It does seem sensible and hard to object to, and many should participate. It seems accountable and democratic, it invites knowledge and participation, it counts as an example of really accomplishing something, and it is defined as a new and inclusive arena for important discussions. All in all, these are self-evident justifications.

In an idealized and perfect bureaucracy (Weber 1978:956-1005), meetings would be unnecessary because everybody would know what to do according to given rules and regulations. In this light, frequent meetings and ideas about indispensable benefits coming from meetings suggest anything but a perfect bureaucracy in today's organizations. We include both meetings and documents in the administrative tasks we aim to investigate in this book because they are often contrasted to hands-on activities or "core activities" in a profession: for example, education when it comes to teachers, treating patients when it comes to nurses and doctors, interacting with clients and their relatives when it comes to social workers, and investigating or patrolling when it comes to the police. We are interested in the social character and conditions for those meetings where professionals gather to sort out the staff schedules, discuss a new routine, collaborate with other organizations, or take part in the monthly workplace issues. We are especially interested in all of the documentation that goes along with such gatherings—i.e., those ongoing regulating activities that people innovate, cultivate, and spread in organizations that already *are* regulated, often in quite a detailed manner.

Momentum and resistance

One way of spinning the administration wheel is, as in the previous example, to use a meeting to set up a new working group with its own meetings. We will soon turn to many others. What these tactics have in common is Simmel's *Eigendynamik*, i.e., more or less autonomous processes of interaction that create their own momentum. There are ambivalences inherent in today's administrative actions that make them repeat themselves, and if they take place in certain cultural environments, they also easily start to multiply.

Fashion provided one of Simmel's (1904/1957) illustrations of such processes. Fashion is driven by people's need to imitate others and conversely by their need to differentiate. People want to dress in "the latest" way, imitating what is deemed *avant garde* in terms of style and trends, and in doing so, they spread the very fashion they copy. As soon as something has been generally adopted, it can hardly be described as fashion anymore because its growth undermines diversity. Imitation will then be replaced by innovation, and then imitation will rise anew, and so on. The two poles of fashion—imitation at one origin point and innovation at the other—unleash a process that continues indefinitely because the tension between them is basically irresolvable. Within a suitable setting—in Simmel's view, the money economy and the city—the cyclical process of fashion takes off and takes its hold on people. In modern times, fashion expands and proliferates (Simmel 1904/1957, 1978; Nedelmann 1990:251).

Transferred to the administration society, there is an equivalent *Eigendynamik*, we argue, or "construction–destruction mechanism" (Nedelmann 1990:254) that reproduces the very constellation that initiated the original momentum. People in organizations want order, yes, but they also want freedom. The more ambivalences become an integral part of the fabric of society, the greater opportunities will be for the initiation of eigendynamic (autonomous) processes. Democracy is highly valued, and people want to have a say, accepting workplace meetings but not endless meetings. They also want decisions and formal rules, but these may be opposed or offer some leeway, leading to new workplace discussions. The combination of high formality and high variability that breeds eigendynamic is characteristic of modern societies in general (Nedelmann 1990).

People want to structure things carefully and coordinate them with others, but they also want space to maneuver independently and solve things more spontaneously. A step in one direction creates a pressure towards the other, which in turn creates a pressure toward the first, and on and on, like a pendulum movement. Suggestions of a working group or a checklist represent efforts to achieve organizational clarity, transparency, and coordination—i.e., orderliness—but they also entail more or less vague formulations of things yet to be ordered. Emerging and unforeseeable ambiguity will stimulate further administration as a way to, for example, sort out the new things. Within an opportune setting, which is characterized in our study by strong belief in rationality and broadened participation among members of the organization, the cyclical process of administration gains energy and a hold on people and their activities.

In this book, we analyze this process in terms of its moral, emotional, and somewhat magical aspects, i.e., the enchanting and seemingly marvelously transforming qualities of administration (cf. Mauss 2001). When we borrow

Simmel's concept and try to specify it with the help of ethnographic data from a variety of settings, we find moral as well as emotional attractions in doing and expanding administration, along with emotional rewards related to "magic" or enchantment in the results, as we detail in Chapter 5.[1]

Let's return to Lisa in the social services and her ambition to create a checklist, mentioned at the beginning of this introduction. We will stay with her for some time. What happened, in more detail?

Lisa suggested a checklist. There is "nothing" now, she says, that defines what to say to parents when they should be informed about being reported to the social services for maltreatment of their children. Lisa finds it frustrating that there is no predictable order of elements to follow in conducting a preliminary assessment of an incoming case at the social services. Daniel, a colleague, says that it might be hard to define these things "since you never know the content of the talk" and "you have it in your head so to speak, what you've got to include, like a checklist, sort of." Ursula, another colleague, says that everybody has worked with preliminary assessments before, so they are used to it, but such a checklist might facilitate the task for the newly employed.

In the back and forth during the meeting, we note that there was actually a soft but tangible resistance to introducing a checklist because the meeting's participants thought that it was more important for them to be "responsive" and "flexible" vis-à-vis the family. This can be seen as one part of the pendulum movement we described previously. On the other hand, they also agreed that they often ask about many of the same things when meeting new families, such as items related to risk analysis. When the new task seems to revolve around children at risk for experiencing violence, it is important to ask about that, Lisa's colleagues say. However, the cases they encounter are so different from each other that it does not seem wise to use the same checklist for each of them.

Lisa suggests that maybe they are using a model already, the so-called BBIC, assessment tool and its "risk and protection" part (BBIC is a framework for assessment, planning, and reviewing in child welfare in Sweden). Well, no, the others say. They claim to work according to the particular report at hand, and although sometimes BBIC is relevant, sometimes it is not. Ursula says that she always puts questions about the family's networks and resources within networks—that doing so is kind of a routine *for her*. Daniel says, "Yeah, you have a sort of list in your head, but you never know exactly where they are [the families], so you'll have to adapt."

Lisa asks again whether they have discussed the need for an "assessment instrument" in any way, but she does not get overwhelmingly enthusiastic support. Such a tool would be too comprehensive, the meeting participants say. It would take too long to fill out "all these questions" and would perhaps even block a process that already may run quickly and smoothly. "We're not supposed to do a mini-investigation," somebody says, resisting the suggested constraints on one's professional freedom. On the other hand, Ursula notes, the law states that they should start an investigation without further delay, and when they start talking with the family, it already has been decided that the family needs help and support.

So, Lisa's suggestion of a checklist does not gain immediate support. It would be too formalistic with a list of items, even though some things recur all the time. They can manage without lists! This example emphasizes that we cannot say that the administration society always reproduces itself effortlessly or without hesitation. If we analyze a meeting like Lisa's at the social services in Sweden, there seems to be a pendulum movement between her suggestions of "more order" and "administrative control" and the contrasting appeals to professional knowledge, flexibility, and meeting clients "where they are."

As we stated in the beginning of this chapter, however, the administration society does not expand with a dramatic boom. Rather, it does so subtly and discreetly, step by step, when people are trying to do their work. At the very end of this meeting, the discussion tilts in the administrative direction. Ursula's remark about the law and the fact that families should be investigated seems to have had an effect. Now the meeting's participants start talking about a less comprehensive instrument to use, a short one (like the "instrument KAOS"). "*That* would suit us," one participant says. "*That's* the kind of form we like, it only has a couple of tick boxes!"

Lisa responds that if they do not "believe in it," they should not write it up. They are not using this instrument today, are they? she asks. Ursula replies that "basically, we're negative to using these ready-made forms with 108 questions or whatever"—repeating the criticism previously formulated in the meeting—"but we will discuss this again at another meeting and then we will state that we can consider some of the more simple, smaller variants."

What does this mean? It means an almost inconspicuous victory of the administration society, in fact a victory arising from criticism of it. It means new meetings with administrative tasks on the table, and it means that a "smaller variant" of a checklist *will* be introduced and incorporated into the social work—even by actors who initially displayed skepticism.

Here we have what we mean by today's *Eigendynamik* of the administration society. There seems to be an inherent momentum unleashed during a meeting like this, founded on the irresolvable tension between orderliness and improvization, between formulated and tacit structures. A suggestion of a checklist and a reference to the law represent the former, and a series of reminders of "what staff have in their heads" represents the latter. Lisa—herself a proponent of a more textualized order and more administrative rigidity within the social services—situationally took the roles of the others by underlining that if they did not "believe" in it, they should not feel forced to support it, as if dramatizing the ambivalence in just a couple of sentences.

But eventually they did believe in it. Almost everybody does today. It is hard to intervene in the *Eigendynamik* of administration, and it is much easier to spiral along with it.

An ethnographic approach to "doing administration"

The administration society is present in people's everyday lives in both tangible and subtle ways. In spite of this, people's participation in meetings and their reading and production of documents are often overlooked in studies of human services organizations (Åkerström and Jacobsson 2019). Administration not only occupies schedules and calendars, routines, and daily errands but also finds its way into people's identities, emotions, and minds. To set up yet another meeting, to create another document, to email colleagues once again (and cc their colleagues), to make charts and tables in beautiful colors to be presented in future meetings—such practices have become a self-evident way to solve an expanding number of responsibilities and concerns in today's society, almost regardless of what the organization formally does. A growing part of the work time for employees in contemporary companies and organizations goes to administrative practices (Forsell and Ivarsson Westerberg 2014; van Vree 2011).

Researchers point out expanding demands from documentation, accounting, evidence, and evaluations, which easily set other activities aside. What many still define as "core activities"— including to interact with and help the client, to listen to and treat the patient, to provide the customer with service and the student with education—is pushed to the margins (Forsell and Ivarsson Westerberg 2014).[2] In this book, through examples from our ethnographic studies in mainly Swedish human services organizations—the social services, health care, psychiatric care, youth care, the border police (see appendix)—we illuminate and elaborate on how this marginalization is accomplished. In our initial example concerning the checklist, we saw how participants used the meeting time in discussing this list, and we got an indication that more time will go to constructing and discussing it during upcoming meetings. Time is limited, and when administrative tasks are stretched out in such a way, less time remains in the calendar for other tasks, including those that should be viewed as central.

Managers or employees may wish to change the state of affairs, as one director of a detention home remarked to us. But, she explained, cutting down on meetings to free staff to spend more time with clients would involve new meetings, where some will protest. So, for the time being, such efforts have not been realized.

A series of co-varying factors are said to contribute to this development. In the public sector, new governing, control, and management mechanisms are in the limelight: *New Public Management* (Hood 1991), the *Audit Society* (Power 1997), the *evidence movement* (Bohlin and Sager 2011), and the *administration society* (Forsell and Ivarsson Westerberg 2014). Organizations are said to transform and "get distracted" because of the pressure from political, economic, and ideological forces, forcing them to devote an ever-expanding amount of time and energy to countless administrative tasks. There is a quite dominating top-down perspective among researchers in this field who portray workplaces, their managers, and employees as more or less vulnerable victims of far-reaching processes coming from elsewhere and invading these settings, and many employees themselves share this feeling. Researchers who do acknowledge the limitations of a top-down approach tend to study people's counter-strategies, shop-front activities, manipulations, shortcuts, and the like, i.e., their reactions and adjustments, their "lives under pressure" (Bruno et al. 2014; Hjärpe 2019; Lauri 2016; O'Malley et al. 1997).

In this book, we present another, complementary perspective. We do not dismiss all top-down or external explanations, but we want to show how today's expanding administration tendencies *also* can be inferred from an internal or bottom-up *Eigendynamik* in Simmel's perspective. To "do administration"—to engage in the self-multiplying circus of meetings, documents, registering, and accounting—involves a self-reinforcing and self-expanding character that we aim to examine in detail. There is a series of chain reactions within the administration society of today, and a multitude of intricate rewards and attractions that increasingly pull people into administration activities. To "do administration" is not merely burdensome and distracting for those experiencing it on the inside but also socially necessary, appealing, enjoyable, and satisfying—*alternatively* bitter and charming, a pendulum movement between grumbling and rejoicing, as we witnessed in Lisa's checklist meeting. Its practicalities and dynamics, we argue, cannot be depicted simply as resulting from abstract pressures "from above." They also arise from interactions *from within*. Fascinating double-bind relations are being played out, with an emotional and aesthetic magnetism among all of the protocols, meetings, models, and charts that so inescapably seem to define our work activities today.

Our aim in this book is to show how employees in public organizations—especially those formally handling clients or patients of one sort or the other—both engage and become entangled in such self-reinforcing and highly immersive interactions.

Conclusion

In the following chapters, we provide a sociological picture of the administration society as it is "done" and "stretched" in practice—with its peculiar rewards and attractions, formations, tensions, contradictions, and conflicts—and how this practice contributes to its very reproduction and expansion. We have tried not to rely on abstract levels or models and instead sought to use rich examples from ethnographic studies in Sweden. Only by seeing and listening to people in administrative situations—and their attached texts, slide shows, messages, diagrams, plans, and protocols—can we gain new insights into why this rather astonishing success of bureaucratization continues to flourish in people's working lives and conquer more and more of its areas.

In the next chapter, we look at some of the trends that underlie these processes and the factors that drive this ever-expanding administrative spiral.

Notes

1 We are also inspired by Jack Katz (1990, 1999) and his approach to social phenomena when he distinguishes emotional transformations, attractions and repulsion.

2 Brodkin and Majmundar (2010) have drawn attention to yet another consequence of expanding paperwork. They maintain that administratively disadvantaged clients find it too costly to claim eligible welfare services, when "tied up in red tape." The authors found that the goal of case load reduction was reached, but not because of the welfare reform, but because of "administrative exclusion."

2 The administration society

Before we proceed with our analysis in the following chapters, in this chapter we acknowledge some major societal changes that researchers describe as bureaucratic acceleration in many parts of society. This acceleration implies a tendency for employees in various organizations to be occupied by administrative rather than their core tasks. Just like social workers, police officers are said to spend more time with paperwork, doctors do many of the tasks office assistants once did, and teachers must spend more time in meetings and with documentation (e.g., Abramovitz 2005; Baines 2006; Erickson et al. 2017; Forsell and Ivarsson Westerberg 2014). Below, we briefly touch on societal and organizational trends that taken together may explain the increase in administrative tasks: new ways of governing, changing administrative occupations, marketization, democratization and representation, collaboration, and digitalization.

New ways of governing and managing

Two main trends related to governing and managing are often depicted in the literature. The first, based on a comparatively new way of governing, has been labeled *New Public Management*. It describes efforts to use private sector management models to make the public service more "businesslike," customer-friendly, and efficient. Early advocates described this management strategy as something of a "post-bureaucracy," where staff could be freed from the bureaucratic "iron cage" that Max Weber (1958) described. The hope was that this way of managing would enable managers and workers to rely on their own judgment and skills. The result, however, has been to some extent intensification of bureaucracy while various ways of measuring customer satisfaction and efficiency evolved. As Farell and Morris (1999) were already discussing from their studies of doctors, teachers, and social workers some 20 years ago, instead of decreased bureaucratization, more management layers have formed as public institutions have been preoccupied with comparing and auditing developments. Discussing the Nordic welfare states, Askeland and Strauss (2014:245) made similar points 15 years later.

DOI: 10.4324/9781003108436-2

The trend to an increasing number of management layers is associated with a second trend: a widespread audit culture. This tendency of contemporary society was so strong that Michael Power (1997) had, by 1997, already entitled his well-known book *The Audit Society—Rituals of Verification*. He investigated auditing as a principle of social organization and control, designed to monitor and measure performance. More recently, the term has been used to refer to and theorize the emergence of these tendencies within the human services. Auditing leads to a preoccupation with measuring professional activities. Efforts are made to measure results and output in quantifiable terms that demand administrative efforts by human services staff in terms of reporting and documenting their work (Carlstedt and Jacobsson 2017; Hjärpe 2019).

Strongly associated with audit culture in medical and social work is a *quest for evidence* for various treatment or therapy models (Bohlin and Sager 2011; Timmermans and Berg 2003). Different ways of collecting information to identify the best and most efficient treatment have evolved into an "evidence movement" demanding that more scientific disciplines adhere to strict quantitative investigations of various interventions (e.g., Jacobsson and Meeuwisse 2020). When these efforts reach not only medical institutions but also social work units and prisons, for example, the result is demands for documentation.

Various management trends may also encourage administrative work. One such trend, known as Lean, is mostly associated with staff efficiency. This management model has been imported from the car industry into various public organizations, such as hospitals (Radnor et al. 2012). Instead of efficient processing of cars, however, its aim was processing patients in a well-ordered, systematic way. The Lean model included teamwork and daily meetings, often in front of a whiteboard where goals and productivity were visible to all in the team. This model has since been incorporated into not only hospitals, but also into various human services organizations such as preschools (Thedvall 2019) and taken up by social authorities in municipalities that handle child welfare and assistance assessment for the elderly, sick, or disabled (Hjärpe 2020).

In addition to functioning as controllers, today's administrators are preoccupied with externally directed self-presentations because both companies and public organizations should "sell themselves" to sometimes hard-to-please customers and service users (Farrell and Morris 1999). Along with New Public Management came an interest in and competition for customers, which has entailed production of documents and meetings not only to "the market," but also directed "inwards," explaining how to sell one's services. The British sociologist Norman Fairclough (1993) has empirically explored this tendency in relation to discourse, and Swedish researchers (Enell, Gruber, and Vogel 2018:30) have discussed markets in relation to the care of children. In another Swedish study of universities, Agevall and Olofsson (2020:38) found that the number of communicators increased by

475% between 2001 to 2018. According to these authors, this astonishing increase can be framed by the background of the universities' current competitive landscape. They have to sell their institutions both to students and to funding organizations.

Changing occupational landscape

The push for specialization is visible in large organizations with growing numbers of departments, divisions, and units. The number of management positions rises accordingly in the form of the department head, division head, unit leader, and so on.

Parallel to this development is the construction of a structure of new types of occupations associated with management, the "management bureaucrats," according to the political scientist Patrik Hall (2012). The increase in university communicators was mentioned previously, but these bureaucrats also consist of human relations staff, public relations staff, controllers, coordinators, and "support functions," among others. In the public sector in Sweden, these categories have expanded while the numbers of teachers and nurses have decreased (Table 2.1). It is also worth noting the decrease in "other administrative staff," that is, administrative assistants. The work that they did, such as typing, sorting, and documenting, is now done by doctors and teachers (Forsell and Ivarsson Westerberg 2014), or in universities by teachers and researchers, which has made such tasks "organizationally invisible" (Agevall and Olofsson 2020:30).

Many of these new occupations are involved in how to govern and control according to new management ideologies and practices, as well as in launching and introducing new reforms that in turn demand more administrators. To

Table 2.1 From the daily paper *Dagens Nyheter Opinion*, by Patrik Hall September 9, 2017.[1]

Development of staff in the public sector	2001	2013	Change (%)
Managers	34,462	51,452	+49
Administrators, economists, human relations staff, marketing managers	45,771	68,769	+50
Other administrative staff	83,574	64,331	–23
Police officers	15,496	16,930	+9
Educators	168,444	140,046	–17
Psychologists, social workers, etc.	24,983	30,531	+22
Nurses, midwives, and other care staff	468,878	451,293	–4
Public sector, total	1,229,752	1,238,351	+0.7

[1]   https://www.dn.se/debatt/allt-fler-styr-och-kontrollerar-allt-farre-gor-sjalva-jobbet/
Note: *This table contains only numbers for 2001 and 2013 because the method for gathering statistics changed after 2013. However, in Hall's new research project, he has gathered new data from 2008–2019 from Swedish regions and local governments, and they show the same tendency: a steep increase in higher-ranking administrative staff, such as controllers, communicators, human relations staff, etc. (personal communication).*

achieve their ends, these administrators engage in meetings with others, draw up documents, and perform other administrative tasks, in the process involving others in meetings and creating documents. Furthermore, they create meta-levels in that controllers may want to meet other controllers in a large organization, or communicators might not be satisfied with communicating results or news only from their division but want to discuss "communication issues" with other communicators (Hall, Leppänen, and Åkerström 2019).

Furthermore, contemporary moral imperatives may give rise to various management bureaucrats. This level may consist of ethical boards or committees, sustainability efforts, or efforts to correct injustices based on gender, disability, and ethnicity. One article on bureaucracy in North American universities asserted that the tendency to hire "diversity officials" was partly the result of new rules and regulations but to a higher degree was instigated by other administrators.

> … one study found that for every dollar spent to comply with government rules, voluntary spending on bureaucracy totaled $2 at public universities and $3 at private ones. Robert Martin of Centre College in Kentucky, a co-author of the study, says the real reason for the growth in spending is that administrators want to hire subordinates, thereby boosting their own authority and often pay, rather than faculty, over whom they have less power. Bureaucrats outnumber faculty 2:1 at public universities and 2.5:1 at private colleges, double the ratio in the 1970s.
>
> (*The Economist*, 2018/05/08)

Democratization and representation

The socio-historian van Vree (1999, 2011) concludes that the ever-increasing number of meetings began in historical processes where talk and negotiation—from court councils and eventually to parliaments—replaced battles and controlled physical violence. In his analysis of meetings, he sees "parliamentarization" as one important stage in the process toward the "meetingization" of contemporary society.

> While increasingly more people became more strongly tied to individual states with the introduction of national duties, such as military service, tax obligations, compulsory education and obligations to social security, and national systems developed for the registration of the population, jurisdiction, the police, education, social and medical care and social security, the competitive struggle for power, possession, and status within states acquired more the character of a regulated battle of words or a parliamentary struggle.
>
> (van Vree 2011:251)

Indeed, meetings in more modern times have played a significant role in many social movements' efforts to put participatory democracy into practice (e.g., Polletta 2002; Sandler 2011). In this context, meetings may be interpreted as part of a political ideal of openness and participation, which is also evident in, for example, directives of the presence of a union ombudsman in negotiations over the closing of a company and student representation at the university board. The democratization process is also visible in non-formal demands for representation. Less explicit but clearly supported by strong norms is the anchoring process that managers engage in to "get all aboard" when new policies, projects, or changes are introduced into workplaces.

Collaboration

According to van Vree's (2011) account for the "meetingization" of contemporary societies, democratization is an important part of societal changes in terms of a larger number of people becoming mutually dependent on each other. The need for coordination is fed by organizations' increasing cooperation with each other, which demands more coordination, and coordination often demands more meetings, and meetings are often integrated with documents. This complexity increases with the quest for collaboration.

Collaboration is now highly desired within public agencies: a tendency shaped by deficits arising from too much specialization. A young delinquent is not only punished by social control agencies but also is seen to need psychological rehabilitation and school counseling, and he may find that his juvenile home contact person confers with the school representative as well as his psychologist and his social worker. Sometimes, however, collaboration may take place for less obvious reasons, as if it has a value of its own—it is *the* cherished work method. An article published in *Harvard Business Review* with the title "Collaborative Overload" illustrates the administrative expansion that may result from exhortations to collaborate:

> Collaboration is taking over the workplace. — teamwork is seen as a key to organizational success. According to data we have collected over the past two decades, the time spent by managers and employees in collaborative activities has ballooned by 50% or more. /.../ Consider a typical week in your own organization. How much time do people spend in meetings, on the phone, and responding to e-mails? At many companies, the proportion hovers around 80%, leaving employees little time for all the critical work they must complete on their own. Performance suffers as they are buried under an avalanche of requests for input or advice, access to resources, or attendance at a meeting.
>
> (Cross et al. 2016)

Digitalization

The trust in and hopes for efficiency in digitalization of the public sector are far-reaching. One example is the Swedish governmental report, "By using the possibilities of digitization the government can increase efficiency in operations and quality for users" (SOU 2016:89, p. 158). But technological changes have paved the way for a radical digitalization of practically all tasks that administrative assistants previously performed manually: ordering travel tickets, arranging schedules, writing letters, and taking routine notes. Now the professionals themselves are supposed to master demanding digital administrative systems. This re-organization of the division of labor has indeed reduced the number of administrative assistants. According to an interview about an ongoing research project with researcher Anders Ivarsson Westerberg, several hundred thousand people occupied these positions in Sweden only 25 years ago, whereas now there are about 30,000.[1]

Research in contexts as diverse as the Swedish police (Ivarsson Westerberg 2004), Australian university teachers (Anderson 2006), and Swedish universities (Agevall and Olofsson 2020) indicates that today, less time is spent on core activities. This contraction is quite often explained by digitalization, and criticism is disseminated via the mass media, such as a series of articles in a Swedish daily, when a headmaster reported that he had 25 different digital systems that do not "work with each other."[2] Below is an illustration from such complaints in relation to digital tasks. This is from a workplace diary that a researcher at a Swedish university shared with us:

> Today I had a lot of work in front of a computer with the support of various communication tools or systems (Agresso, the schematic system, university internal web for support and documents, Skype). The work with data files in research projects involves a support contact with the company that provides software and their subcontractor of training in the software. I have had this contact for about one year and have not yet received a data file that works to work in. Even the IT help desk at the university has been / are involved when it comes to how the file should be managed on my computer and on the university network. Today I (which I often do) lack a clearer support regarding administration and finances where different people undertake to solve tasks and instead I get a lot of tasks to solve in order for them to solve their task. --- Both yesterday and today, it felt like as if I was working in the HR department first, then the economy division, then the "marketing division" with the task of processing and handling external inquiries, in the university management and "the internal support department for questions about everything." Often, working days can also include work in the communications department and IT help desk so as not to forget the student service department and janitorial staff.

Digitalization has provided organizations with opportunities and demands to document one's work, to fill in orders, to report exams, to create journals, etc. This documentation work is often placed with staff whose core occupation is defined by other tasks which implies that staff complain about "low clerical work and accountability requirements"; sometimes such criticism derives from complaints about time spent on what is pejoratively termed "bright ideas" emanating from middle management level, according to Gina Anderson (2006:584).

Rhetorical critique dressed in numbers

This chapter gives an overview of social and organizational trends associated with increased administrative engagements, efforts, and tasks. We close by pointing out that many of the illustrations used to demonstrate what is seen as excessive administration rely on the magic of numbers because doing so is rhetorically efficient. When *The Economist* (as quoted above) reports that "Bureaucrats outnumber faculty 2:1 at public universities and 2.5:1 at private colleges, double the ratio in the 1970s," it both offers an example of the changing occupational landscape of many organizations and makes rhetorical points. The numbers aim at appealing both to our sense that universities ought to be populated by researchers and teachers rather than bureaucrats, and that this is not a given: not too long ago (1970s), the situation was quite different. Such implicit argumentation with numbers may be convincing because "numbers seem to be 'hard facts'—little nuggets of indisputable truth" (Best 2012:17).

If we look at a few more examples that are relevant to the current criticism, which often focuses on what is seen as an overload in relation to professions and the numbers presented in research, different evaluations and debates have an important role in various arguments. One such case was, at first glance, a bit surprising. Two chief physicians commented on the much-debated contemporary problems in health care, such as long queues, postponed surgeries, and staff shortages. In contrast to the common demands for more resources for health care, these physicians argued against this solution in a debate article in a large Swedish daily with the heading, "Extra funding feeds an unstoppable bureaucracy":

> We suggest that one starts with a critical examination of how the health care sector uses its time, staff, and other resources. 2014 was the first year that administrative staff in the health care sector exceeded the number of doctors—and that development continues. Health care regions have large teams of communicators, not unusual with 50–100 employees in a medium-sized region.[3]

As with the ratio of administrative staff and faculty at universities, the ratio of administrative staff and doctors can be put forward to foster moral indignation. The specification of the year 2014 further emphasizes the correctness of the claim that administrators from this point in time actually outnumber the doctors. Anything but the exact range of 50–100 employees is still better rhetorically than vaguely formulating this as, for instance, "many communicators."

Another illustration comes from the social services sector: the claim that social workers meet children with whom they are supposed to work for only 2% of their working hours. The number derives from a Swedish report written by a civil servant whom the government commissioned to evaluate child welfare investigations and suggest policy changes (*Barnets och ungdomens reform* 2017:47). The phrase "Only 2% time with the children" has been repeated and used widely in the media and by the government, unions, and local authorities to argue against a growing bureaucratization of the social services or legitimizing more resources to this sector (Hjärpe 2020). Social scientists who are critical about the state of affairs can also use such information, enhancing the implications of these numbers. For example, Swedish organizational researcher Mats Alvesson (2019:16) picked up the 2% and converted that value into "ten minutes a day" in a recent book, thus joining the chorus of critique against bureaucratic growth that nowadays are rather mainstream.

Although evidence points to a growing administration in general, as we have discussed previously, it is important to note that some of the same statistics can be highlighted for rhetorical purposes by actors who are skeptical or deeply critical of this trend. Statistics lend themselves to such influences (Best 2012).

Conclusion

In this chapter, we have highlighted major social and organizational trends that have been argued to underlie bureaucratic acceleration in new arenas. These tendencies have involved new approaches to governing, marketization in institutions that previously focused less on marketing needs, the seeping of the "quest for evidence" into medical-adjacent organizations, collaboration, the growing management class and accompanying changes in administrative occupations, democratization, and digitalization. We also emphasized how numbers can be used as a form of rhetorical sleight of hand to support claims about a far too excessive bureaucracy. In the next chapter, we look at why, despite the critiques that these numbers sometimes serve to support, participants can find administrative tasks attractive and even seductive, rather than burdensome.

Notes

1 *Skolvärlden*, 4 maj, 2016. "Lärare lägger 50 procent på administration." [Teachers spend 50% on administration.] https://skolvarlden.se/artiklar/forskning-visar-larare-lagger-50-procent-pa-administration
2 The Swedish daily *Sydsvenskan* 2020-06-12.
3 https://www.svd.se/extrapengar-goder-en-ostoppbar-byrakrati

3 Seductive gatherings

Meetings often express authority and hierarchy, and managers, bureaucrats, and employees use them as an arena to formulate policies and execute power. But there is also a common critique of meetings as tedious and meaningless. A large collection of studies by Allen and colleagues, *The Cambridge Handbook of Meeting Science* (2015), reflects meeting critique in contemporary working life and mentions "meeting fatigue" (Kello 2015) and "meeting burnout" (Olien et al. 2015:17) among future research questions worthy of exploration. A study of Swedish managers showed that half of their meetings were seen as meaningless.[1] Still, a meeting holds some appeal as an event that pulls its participants together, making them pay attention to concerns presented as crucial and shared, with careful monitoring for any effort to escape from these concerns, followed by booking new, upcoming meetings in what today seems to be never-ending chains.

A meeting combines sense and nonsense, drama and dullness. It is a phenomenon characterized by sociological ambivalence (Merton 1976), since it artfully merges normative and liberating features. It creates a special aura of both plight and pleasure. Its participants are driven not only to engage in its emerging discussions but also to return to the subsequent gathering, despite having been bored by the formalities the last time. Sometimes people sigh over the burden of being in a meeting, but they may also imagine beforehand with anticipation (and in detail) what to say or regret afterwards what they did not say but thought about. In any case, the pull is evident. In many organizations, a meeting can be "*the* place to 'be seen and be heard,'" as Schwartzman (1989:125) puts it, a sort of ritual site for where "the action" is (Goffman 1967/1982:149–270), a place to show one's competence, have one's character tested, make relations clear, and win or lose local battles.

The attraction of meetings is not contrary to critique against bureaucratization and organizational rigidity but parallel to it. It coexists with the critique, so that a sigh over time-consuming meetings quickly can be exchanged with effervescence and enthusiasm. Consider, for instance, this situation from a youth care institution, when Nellie, heading for the conference room, meets Laura, her colleague:

DOI: 10.4324/9781003108436-3

Laura asks what Nellie is heading to now, and Nellie sighs and rolls her eyes. She nods at all of the papers and folders she is holding in her hands and says, "it's just one of those monthly meetings." "But I heard *you* had done such an interesting excursion!" Laura starts asking Nellie about her latest work, and now I'm passing them on the stairs. I [the ethnographer] get the impression that Laura does not want to talk about the upcoming meeting at all, but prefers to talk about more exciting things in Nellie's work, instead. They all revolve around other things than meetings.

Later on, when the meeting has started, Nellie turns out to be one of the most engaged participants. She does not sit quietly, just waiting for the meeting to be over. She is sharply commenting on the issues, contributing with suggestions, and delivers jokes and sarcasm. She is using a lot of gestures to entertain the others. And they laugh, so she succeeds. She elaborates on the agenda during the meeting, and she brings in new aspects. She is really engaged in the meeting.

What social forces are at work that lead someone like Nellie to be so nonchalant at first and so engaged later?

A meeting is a carefully regulated gathering, tying its participants to a certain room at a certain time of day, holding them within certain topics that are to be debated with a certain vocabulary and style—or with careful steps marking how the expected vocabulary and style are temporarily suspended. A meeting may actually hold its members so tight to its concerns that they develop tailored techniques to manipulate or get around it, survive within it, or make it proceed more according to their wishes. These techniques also keep the spiral of meetings running. They ensure that people stand the burden and get something out of it. Today's administration society (Forsell and Ivarsson Westerberg 2014) is far from being characterized only by highly engaging meetings; there are also a lot of boring ones. In our data, these aspects do not contrast but interfold with and feed each other.

In this chapter, we show the social effervescence of the very activity of having a meeting and how the social control of the meeting society is re-produced and managed. Meetings, we argue, provide a captivating frame for people's work-related interactions that easily gain their own momentum by continually shifting between formal and informal, seriousness and playful-ness, and control and escape-the-control. This back-and-forth renewing of momentum is the overarching theme of this chapter, and these pendulum swings play a crucial role when today's administration society turns eigendynamic (Nedelmann 1990:244).

Meetings are particularly attractive in settings where ideas of rationality and participation are celebrated, and where, for that reason, they are attributed high status. They are typically seen as a forum for important decisions and a way for "all" to contribute, a place for democratization, but what happens in practice may very well be another story.[2] Things other than important decisions take place in meetings, too, and not "all" contribute.

The fact that a meeting easily attracts and even engrosses its participants is striking in our data. In many instances, individuals may on one occasion fervently participate in a discussion of an apparently very engaging topic, but on a later occasion drop their engagement and the topic, never raising the issue again. One of us followed the type of meeting that Nellie attended at a youth care institution (in the above excerpt) and noted how Nellie and her colleagues engaged with various topics and concerns on youth care issues that later on seemed to have been quite forgotten, replaced by other topics and concerns.

Meetings thus seem to be arenas where the involvement is *situationally sustained*, which may transform or cease with changing circumstances. Schwartzman (1989:164–165) describes this fluctuating involvement:

> … people would move on to new meetings, frequently appearing to forget the issues that only last week had seemed to be life-and-death struggles. For example, the activities of one particular Drug Abuse Task Force were followed for one year. This group met every week and included center staff as participants as well as individuals from other agencies in the community. These meetings were characterized by long and sometimes very bitter debates about proper service modalities. Eventually, this group decided to write a proposal to secure funds to coordinate drug abuse services for the West Park area. At the end of a year, the proposal was completed after a long and very complex negotiation process. Shortly thereafter and much to the researcher's surprise, the proposal was lost, and even more remarkable was the fact that no one seemed to notice or care.
>
> (Schwartzman 1989:164–165)

The remarkable and transformative power of meetings is, in other words, a reason to investigate their situational structure, its variations and practices, and people's ways of becoming mesmerized by it, using it, and manipulating it.

Into the meeting form

A meeting typically brings people together and creates the opportunity for them to generate and comment on their relationships with each other: people "move from one form of interaction (chats, two-party discussions, etc.) into the meeting form" (Schwartzman 1989:125). A subtle framing process occurs, tightening up the interactions and streamlining people's postures and emotions. Members start to attend to the agenda, they compose themselves a bit and display their version of a *meeting persona*, convincingly communicating that they will—basically—stay like this until a set of important things is addressed, discussed, or solved. Order is attributed to the chairperson, who directs the talk.

To "strike the tone" and begin a meeting—to situationally accomplish the meeting frame—is important. The chairs may, for instance, take a seat, arrange papers, clear their throat, sweep with a gaze to the others in the room, and say things like "okay, let's start" or "well, shall we get started?" (Atkinson, Cuff and Lee 1978). Certain phrases, gestures, movements, and gazes are used to remind people of why they are there and to phase out other activities. In our data, we find plenty of examples of mundane but significant cues and markers that in various ways indicate that a meeting is starting.[3]

> There are some minutes left until the meeting will start. Carolyn [the principal] sits in front of me [the ethnographer] at the "wrong" end of the conference table, explaining the so-called process map for detention homes. The teachers have dropped in, all in all 12 men and women, and taken their seats and are putting their calendars, pens, notebooks, cell phones, and institutional alarms at the table. They chat. Next to one teacher, there is a packet of cigarettes. In the middle, there is a coffee thermos and some mugs.

> Carolyn takes her time and finishes her talk with me. Then she closes the binder [containing the process map] and returns to her ordinary chairperson position at the other short end of the table. Now she sits at the "right" place. People soon stop chatting, straighten up a bit, and turn towards Carolyn. "Well," she says, "shall we get started?" It is not a question, I [the ethnographer] think to myself; it is the start.

A meeting's social control is seamlessly integrated into how the actors establish and sustain its recognizable frame. It would be tempting to see Carolyn, the principal in the above-quoted excerpt, as solely "doing" this frame as she closes the binder and returns to her chairperson position at the conference table, saying, "shall we get started?", but in fact the other teachers—her colleagues—are involved in the accomplishment as well. They subtly observe Carolyn's position in the room, they relate somehow to her movement from one end of the table to the other, and they anticipate her mundane call for order by silencing before she starts, thereby contributing to the meeting frame. It is not Carolyn on her own who makes sure that people are brought together and moved from one form of interaction into the meeting form (Schwartzman 1989:125)—the meeting members collectively do so.

As they drop into the conference room before the meeting, they communicate a culturally shared understanding of what a meeting is and why it is important. They have brought their meeting props (pens, papers, laptops, and coffee), they take their seats, they engage in interactions of a brief, trivial, and conspicuously interruptible type (chatting, trivia talk), implicitly signaling "just some minutes left," "what we do now will soon evaporate," and "we just wait for the *real* thing to begin" (Yoerger, Francis and Allen 2015). They attend to what their chair is doing and where she is. They act as if situated in a kind of meeting prologue. Carolyn just has to pull the trigger, so to speak: "Well, shall we get started?"

These patterns of subtle adaptations and discreet use of cultural resources within organizations are mobilized in the administration society's *Eigendynamik*. When new meetings are proposed and when established meetings expand and become even more morally honored and respected, members of an organization today typically know exactly how to behave. A meeting seldom requires an explanation, in its entirety or in its details. You just need to say, "I'm busy, away for a meeting." Nobody asks about the goal of the meeting or why it is necessary to attend. The frame is highly re-cognizable and basically invokable at any time, and in today's organizations, it has become very attractive.

A meeting is a perfect form for displaying relations in an organization. Schwartzman (1989: 128) argues that social relations "acted out" in a meeting are legitimized, including possible conflicts, because they are con-sidered to be "the business" of the organization. She also notes that when people converge on a specific place at a specific time, the times surrounding the start and finish (as well as breaks) assume great importance (Schwartzman 1989:124). Members of a given organization now get the opportunity to exchange gossip, engage in shop talk, trade information, or hold "pre-meetings" to prepare their team performance (Yoerger, Francis and Allen 2015). How people manage the surrounding times in relation to a meeting is in itself meaningful. Who arrives with whom, who chats with whom, who is early and who is late, who sits all alone, who is so important that the meeting cannot start without her—people's arrivals and departures, postures, and facial expressions can be highly significant for communicating status, alliance, support, or opposition (Schwartzman 1989: 284).

We have touched on how the meeting frame is clarified—from small talk to proper formal meetings by the chair, and how participants may use pre-meetings. Ending a meeting also includes its ritualistic bridging. The chair may formally declare the meeting's end. If the meeting collects people from the same workplace, the chair may ease the bridge by reminding the par-ticipants that they soon will see each other for coffee or for lunch. If the meeting is not one of many in an already set schedule (such as "the Tuesday meeting"), many meetings end with the participants or some of them en-gaged in arranging a new meeting. They take their calendars and try to find a new time, one of the many versions in which the meeting *Eigendynamik* is illustrated.

The meeting as an arena for displayed social relations and positionings contributes to its popularity. Meetings make organizations visible and tan-gible for their members (Hall, Leppänen and Åkerström 2019), which can be especially crucial amidst the many abstract and hard-to-explain work tasks in today's society. The most meeting-intensive areas in the settings we have studied are also those that are most engaged in abstract issues, the discursive or representational issues of how this or that should be displayed, reported, and talked about—and how symbolization should work. We may expect that the drive for meetings is most articulated here, and we may also expect many meetings when organizational members are striving to *transform* concrete tasks into abstract ones. As we show in the example below, there is an attraction in fleeing from clients and doing abstractions.

In a project within Swedish youth care that we followed (Åkerström 2019), a new group of coordinators was supposed to develop a "client-near" working style, a style that was never really explained in concrete terms. The new coordinators came to be surrounded by an aura of having a very important mission, but exactly what that mission was remained unclear. Quite soon, they ended up working in a conspicuously meeting-bureaucratic way. Instead of focusing on getting in touch with the young people directly and moving forward with their work of helping them with, for instance, medical treatment, new apartments, missing school assignments, job opportunities, drug problems, and family relations, the coordinators spent much of their time in meetings with other officials—and other coordinators. Talking *about* the clients turned out to be easier than talking *with* them, and scheduling one's work according to an office logic was much easier than improvised and tailored social work with a group of young people with experiences of criminality, drug use, and other morally ambiguous activities in the societal margins.

In this environment—with (at least sometimes) restless young people and meeting-oriented officials—the coordination project was launched. The coordinators did not want to work in a meeting-less void, trying to get in contact with clients without having a recognizable frame for it, like the social services' fieldworkers would, for instance (so-called *fältare* in Swedish). They wanted agendas and coffee, meeting chairs and written protocols, meeting tables, and meeting times. They preferred to clarify their work in terms of relations to other professionals and to other coordinators, in and through documents and meetings, rather than cultivating relations with the young people directly. They even used the new project to invent a plethora of new types of meetings within Swedish youth care.

Stiff and relaxed

What seems to be characterizing meetings within organizations today is their particular combination of formalities and informalities. The teacher meetings that we observed in a detention home, for instance, elegantly alternated between a range of important discussions, messages, and updates on teaching and institutional matters (including individual pupils and their status), and jokes, personal praise, storytelling, sarcasm, fun insinuations, and critique.[4] What is captivating with the meeting frame in our studies is, at closer inspection, not to be found only within its formalities but also next to them.[5] Meeting members drift back and forth in relation to the meeting frame. Local cultures and different meetings seem to supply accountable behavioral codes for their members to alternate between layers of constraint and liberation, so that an interest in what is happening—the action, in Goffman's (1967/1982:149–270) terms—can be continually sustained.

In our data, we can see how these and other alterations build up a considerable part of the meeting's attractive power. It would not be fair to say that formalities reign as soon as the chair clears her throat and says, "Well, shall we get started?" (Atkinson et al. 1978), only to be dissolved when the meeting ends. Rather, many meetings are filled with glimpses or periods of informalities within the proceedings. To an outside observer, the meeting may be quite formal and stiff on the surface, but an observer who moves closer to the participants may see how they exchange ironic notes (but with a straight face). In other meetings, participants may be allowed to continually bracket the formal frame and insert their jokes, ironies, and entertaining comments, charging the meeting with energy by using frames within a frame.

One such type of meeting exemplified in our interviews with chairs at university departments was the management team meeting. These meetings were described by a former manager as "therapeutic," and the administrator cited below describes these meetings through the metaphor of a "valve" (in Swedish: *ventil*). When asked whether some meetings could be fun, he answered:

> The management team. We handle very different things of different kinds. But we're actually trying to have fun. And it's a little bit 'cause it's supposed to be a valve [Swedish: *ventil*]. So, you have to joke together — we use each other in that way. But also, we must be allowed to laugh. We can have some fun. If someone stands in the corridor outside they may wonder what we are doing ... 'Cause there're so many meetings you've got to hold so formally. Still, we've a lot of things to deal with, but we can do it in a way that feels easier.

The chair compared these meetings with board meetings, which he believed have—and must have—a more formal setting with an agenda. Furthermore, however:

> ... in the management group we have to trust each other one hundred percent. What's said in here, it's said in here. And I really don't feel that security in relation to the board. Actually. And that also matters.

Such contrasts are often used when managers describe their different meetings. A manager at a detention home talked about how much he liked therapy sessions with families. He contrasted these sessions to meetings about administering the organization, which were described as being a "bit boring." The therapy sessions, on the other hand, were "exciting meetings." These were "breathtaking, fun ones, you can go on and on," and during these he was "extremely focused." Another manager at a detention home mentioned that he appreciated meetings where he met colleagues who were also managers from other parts of youth care. These meetings offered some change and an opportunity to meet new people. For him, these are events:

> … that we look forward to, because then you meet a lot: Both people you know a little bit, and other, external people who are in it, that … and it always feels fun. A bit new. /…/ 'cause it's always more of the same with the other meetings.

Attending to administrative concerns may imply going about one's business in a partly formal or "stiff" way. Had we been at the meetings described above—the chair's board meeting or the ordinary meetings of the managers of detention homes—we might still have had some glimpses of fun. Having fun, at least in parts of the meeting, keeps up participants' attention and makes them enjoy this type of social gathering because they constantly can watch, enjoy, and analyze potential frame shifting. The captivating quality of the meeting frame not only rests in its being culturally recognizable, invokable at many times and for multiple purposes, and thus "safe" as a working form, but also in its potential to harbor other frames within the frame, which the participants must navigate. A vivid meeting is, in that sense, at least a little unpredictable.

The meetings that Schwartzman (1989:134) observed in a mental health center in the 1970s became explicitly emotional and conflicting. A "good meeting" from the participants' perspectives actually involved "a great deal of emotion, expressions of conflict, crying, posturing, yelling, and so forth." When discussions turned less emotional and more formal at the health center, staff could see this as a way to deny or suppress feelings. Meetings in our data are less emotional than in Schwartzman's study but nevertheless are characterized by shifting grades of formality and emotionality. Joking, playfulness, irony, "putting on a character," and similar maneuvers turned out to be a substantial aspect of participants' framework in and around many meetings in our data, as well, and something that maintained people's interest (cf. Schwartzman 1989:301).

In our data from detention homes, in the beginning of a teachers' meeting, a turn to speak was given to Olle, a teacher engaged as a safety representative. He, in turn, had just been to another meeting where he was reprimanded about teachers at the detention home reporting too few in-cidents of violence within the institution compared to treatment staff. The security group wanted the teachers to report more cases, he was told. "Why is there never anyone from the school reporting?" Even though the school constitutes a "good working environment" (minimizing risks for violence), this cannot be the only explanation, Olle says. There must be incidents not reported, and the teachers—now assembled at this meeting—are the ones who should be reporting. Olle gives this information in an extended and sharp way during the teachers' meeting, as if forwarding the reprimand he got himself at the meeting before.

> Olle talks energetically about the importance of making teachers report more, and he mentions many examples. Once, for instance, when "five girls were put down" [by staff during a physical fight] at a ward, there was no report. "Then *you* were there," Olle says, nodding at Dave, the new coordinator between school and wards.

> "No," Dave says with a straight face, "then it [the violent incident] would never have happened." Many teachers laugh. Ylva smiles and says, "You can say that *here!*"

Subsequently, the discussion proceeds in a more serious tone. The teachers talk about the definition of an incident and whether one really should report if a situation de-escalates, for example, so the Dave-and-Olle exchange passes quickly. Nonetheless, it contains a lot. Dave manages to insert an alternative and jocular frame within Olle's basically reprimanding lecture, attracting others' humor and giving them a laugh. He also manages to insert critique against treatment staff who are not present at this meeting. By implying—jokingly—that the situation with the girls would not have resulted in violence at all if he had been there, Dave is indicating that the treatment staff really cannot handle this kind of situation on their own. Teachers, on the other hand, are much better at conflict management, he suggests, and as a coordinator (mediating between teachers and treatment staff), he happily identifies with the teachers. This is a teachers' meeting, so implicitly Dave invokes the collective solidarity and sharpens a shared identity by pointing out another category's (the treatment assistants) incompetence.

Ylva's response—"You can say that *here!*"—points out Dave's position. He is "safe" here, among the teachers, when implicitly criticizing treatment staff, but things would be different among treatment staff and *their* meetings. "There" he would not have been able to say the same. Ylva's comment is fun, too—it jokes with Dave's joke, prolonging and commenting on it at the same time. Nothing stops Olle from continuing his project during the meeting to inform his colleagues about the importance of reporting more violence, so the inserted exchange does not alter the direction of the meeting. Still the participants laugh and enjoy the interlude.

Our data are full of similar inserted passages. They are artfully crafted and placed, often sophisticated and internally joking, like glimpsing islands of escape in a bureaucratic ocean. They attract the participants and provide some kind of breathing space for them, a moment of relief. It *is* important to talk about violence and how to report it at a detention home, as well as problematizing unrecorded incidents—nobody at the meeting is signaling otherwise—but it is *also* fun to mock a competing and absent category of staff (for not being so good at managing violence) and hear a colleague blatantly praise himself at the same time. It is also fun to point out the fact that this colleague certainly does not take any risks by doing so ("You can say that *here!*").

Meetings would not be very engaging if the participants could not produce both the formal, important stuff and the jokes. Another engaging aspect is not knowing *when* seriousness will briefly give way to play and joking, sarcasm, and insinuations. Basically, participants can never be sure—it may happen at any time. It is no coincidence that Schwartzman (1989:301–302) places the theme "play and joking during meetings" under the heading "Maintaining/encouraging interest and participation" in her book on meetings.[6] To use humor to comment on action not only relieves tension but also sustains attention. The meeting turns into a site for minor dramas and organizationally titillating excitements.

Joking and sarcasm

If we look closely at fun exchanges during meetings, it becomes evident that many of them not only bracket the organizational reality but also encompass it. When Ylva in the above excerpt smiles and says, "You can say that *here!*", she refers to the sometimes tense relations between teachers and treatment assistants, so that the joking passage can be understood as mirroring and commenting on these relations. It is a relief to be able to laugh about treatment assistants' presumably less-competent way of dealing with the young people without escalating troubles into violence. Similarly, it is a relief to laugh at the very division between teachers and treatment assistants within the detention home. It is a bracket, but still the organization is very much there.

Similar constructions of commenting fun-in-brackets can be done very quickly in meetings. It is a matter of in-house joking, often sarcastically aimed at something people find irritating or some kind of internal awkwardness or discomfort that binds the organizational members together.

When we followed a manager at a psychiatric unit, we learned that the head manager had repeatedly suggested to division managers that doctors should also attend some of their meetings. The others had been hesitant: "If they have to sit through meetings when we discuss recruiting occupational therapists and such, they'll hit the roof." In general, the managers united in fairly limited, short critical remarks about the doctors—more so than for other categories. One theme concerns the difficulty in involving doctors in meetings or taking responsibility for organizing them. The following fieldnote is collected from a meeting with two managers:

Anders suggests that an assessment team for a joint assessment of the patients at the psychosis unit would be good: "So one assessment can be made instead of patients being sent around in the house," he says. He jokingly adds that referral conferences in psychiatry usually remind him of a recurring episode from the comic book *Asterix*. "When the Romans appoint a legionary to scout the Gauls, everyone finds very intricate excuses for not being able to join, and finally, some poor newcomer who doesn't really grasp what's going on is the one who goes on the mission," he says with a smile. "Yeah," Stefan says, and he also smiles, "everyone looks down."

Another category that provides a "unifying" object of criticism consists of those "above" in the organization. In Sweden, each manager has to hold regular *medarbetarsamtal* (staff appraisals, literally *collegial talks*) with each employee. These talks are rather structured, and a document produced for this purpose contains directions about what to ask and what to note. During a meeting with different division managers at the psychiatric clinic, the head manager tells them that new instructions have been introduced for these talks.

Stefan says that there was actually already good material about this, so he thinks it is unnecessary. The other meeting participants around the table nod. "We've simply been overrun by the administration on this issue, so there's nothing to do about it," adds Stefan. He says he has no experience with the new material, but he hopes that it will work.

[Discussion on upcoming conference]

The meeting begins to end. Stefan says there is a meeting tomorrow when they will, among other things, receive training on the new material for assessment appraisal. He takes up the agenda on the computer. "You're obviously the one who will be teaching us [how to conduct these meetings]," says Julia, and everyone laughs. Stefan also laughs: "Yes! Oh dear, it was more than I knew," he says. He jokingly says that he will be very carefully prepared. "The new material is very advanced, shoe size becomes the decisive criterion," he continues with a smile, and his smile is reciprocated around the table.

The participants comment on the organization—some stuff coming from above, they seem to say, may be unnecessary, but we just have to accept it. Still, the meeting frame clearly allows—mainly—for mocking the central administration by the suggestion of shoe size and for mocking the head manager, who is not quite aware that he probably will be the one in charge of the (unnecessary) education.

Jokes and ironic comments also can be used against other organizations, particularly in relation to collaborating groups. In a treatment team meeting at a detention home, for instance, the participants spend some time joking about social services workers at the municipalities (i.e., outside the detention home) who to the participants' surprise were working in a very engaging way. "What has happened?" a staff member says in an ironic tone. Another staff member gives the example of a social services worker actually "calling them and checking things" regarding a young person at the institution, whereas "nobody" cared before. There is a general merry atmosphere around this, as is clear from the fieldnotes from this meeting. The meeting participants joke about being surprised over the fact that social services workers *actually do their job*.

Meetings may also provide "backstage" opportunities to joke about clients. Another instance during a treatment meeting at the detention home concerns a more brief and sarcastic remark: a participant mentions a young man in treatment who recently started to be truant because he does not fall under the compulsory school attendance anymore:

> This young man is over 18 years old and "realized" this, someone says, after being informed by other young people or staff. "Well, that bloody information," Mary [a teacher] says and smiles slyly. Everybody laughs.

Joan, a teacher at the detention home, and her colleagues want this adolescent to go to school, and part of the meeting deals with trouble creating school motivation, or in other ways activating young people in general during their stay at the detention home. The information that those over age 18 years formally do not have to go to school is therefore troublesome. It demoralizes the collective and legitimizes truancy—which, strictly speaking, is not truancy anymore because older adolescents are free to skip school. Mary's sarcastic comment, in other words, indicates a complex problem looming behind the meeting's topics, but the solution cannot be to hide the information and pretend that all of the residents in the home have to go to school. The members of the organization will have to content themselves with joking about it.

Still, the joke is telling. The phase "that bloody information" says something about the predicament that the staff consider themselves having with the limits of compulsory schooling. It is hard to encourage or motivate schoolwork for young people with criminal experiences without a principle of compulsory attendance behind you. A wishful thought among the adults would be to just hide "that bloody information" and simply make all the young people go to school. When the teachers laugh at Mary's joke, they also comment on their organization and—in a locally unifying and relieving way—use the meeting to point out and make vivid what is peculiar with their work. This episode, of course, was not on the agenda, but it happened during the meeting. It is a fleeting detail being mentioned, a quickly passing aspect, but significant nonetheless.

Speaking freely

Other instances in our meeting data contain expressions and epithets that never, or at least seldom, would appear in formal minutes or documentation of cases. It is common for meeting participants to accomplish distance by injecting a quite loose and informal jargon or local politically incorrect vocabulary into the dominant formal and correct discourse. These incursions, in turn, accomplish interest in the meeting and motivate members to sustain this form of gathering.

As an example, Joan, the teacher at the detention home, talks about a newcomer among the young people during the above-described treatment team meeting. She characterizes him as sentenced for sexual crimes, such as severe rape. He "fits in well," Joan says and smiles a bit, "he is called 'the gentleman.'"

Such a remark would never be put into official documents, such as case book journals or written decisions. Clients are not supposed to be described ironically—a rapist as a "gentleman"—or with cutting remarks. The meeting's normal vocabulary instead is characterized by expressions such as "risk assessment," "problematic," and with "anti-social values" that are within the expected language of staff in a detention home. It is not considered professional to start describing people freely and in everyday terms, but the meeting form in many cases actually allows for several detours and brackets, which contribute to the feeling of action and that "this is the place to be." There is a relatively elastic discursive moral being played out that keeps the participants alert. It is, after all, a bit invigorating to ironically call a rapist "a gentleman" just because such an expression does *not* belong to the formal background expectations in youth care contexts. The continuous oscillation between formalities and informalities allows for interesting remarks and excursions. Again, we see a version of the pendulum swings that create the back-and-forth motions of the administration society.

Similarly, some meeting participants started to talk about young people comparing privileges all the time, typically producing envy within the wards. If somebody gets some extra leisure time, for instance, or an excursion, the other residents on the wards bring that up and complain about not getting the same thing themselves. "They are like small boys," a staff member says and laughs. "They want the same." This, too, could never have been written in this setting. Nobody would be entitled to liken adolescents at a detention home with "small boys" in a formal document or authoritative account, but it is possible to briefly insert these comments into a meeting, as an ironic wink, and then move on in a more serious tone.

In another episode, the participants discuss a young man in treatment who does not care about his school lessons and spends his time watching the news on the Internet instead of doing math. He would need some "motivational talk," it is said. Ylva, the teacher, says jokingly that she is using a "high-arousal approach" in relation to him—that is, she is using firm orders and scolding. This is, formally, the wrong method within the local culture, and simultaneously a play with words. Staff are often supposed to use a "*low*-arousal approach," engaging in *de-escalation* and *avoiding* unnecessary provocations. The approach that Ylva is describing is blatantly oppositional and implicitly mocking the official line. Still, by saying it jokingly, she can dodge any critique and just go on describing what she is doing at work. Again, the joking tone during the meeting provides a relief and a pause from the formalities and is telling for the organizational realities and the norms at Ylva's workplace. It fits well in the meeting form by displaying the subtle quality of not deviating too much from what is expected, but still inserting a dose of energetic candor.

This momentum between the formal and the informal, we argue, contributes to the attractions of having meetings and going to a meeting. It is hard to convey the same emotions or views in documents or emails, and it is not as fun to read about them as it is to listen to them being improvised and accomplished *in situ*—with a distinct tone of voice, expressive mimicry, and nice timing. Ylva, Joan, and the others can quite safely deliver their brief ironic or sarcastic remarks, and they do so while they are checking the audience's faces and reactions to make sure that nobody will misunderstand them or take what is said literally. In this way, they can perform the daily job of keeping the organization intact and maintaining the working spirit with some extra-moral life. Joking, playfulness, irony, "putting on a character," and similar maneuvers maintain the participants' interest in their daily work (cf. Schwartzman 1989:301).

The meeting form, though, is stable in our data. There are no meetings dissolving into formlessness because of changes in tone or vocabulary, or discussions turning completely joking and playful. Instead, we may argue that the stability of the meeting *gains* from inserted jokes and playfulness, so that a contrast structure helps the meetings to go on. There is a Simmelian tension being built up, creating an eigendynamic motion. If a participant contributes with a comment of more informal and out-of-frame character, the others—and especially the chair—have a clear opportunity to straighten things out in relation to this, as if reconstructing the form with renewed energy and meaning with the help of this relief. In the quotation below, this reconstruction is taking place very subtly, merely in terms of an ironic tone:

> On one occasion, when teachers at a detention home discuss reported violent cases and the importance of taking this seriously, Claude inserts a comment on "ugly words." He is referring to the fact that young people often use a lot of offensive expressions to provoke staff and that they basically can be seen as threatening.

> But Claude says it with an ironic tone, to mark that there must be limits in the demands for reporting. These "ugly words" are abundant in

detention homes, and not everything can be reported. In fact, "ugly words" is an odd term to characterize what staff should look for because they are more or less surrounded by them on a daily basis.

The chair dismisses the comment quickly. "That, you can take," he says promptly. He means that ugly words must be accepted by staff. It is only if the situation as a whole is threatening that one should report. Then he moves on talking in a serious tone, and Claude's comment seems to leave no trace.

"That, you can take"—the chair's reply effectively closes Claude's discreet attempt to ironize, but the attempt is still significant. It functions as a contrast to the seriousness that the meeting form conveys, so that when this seriousness is reconstructed it is done in relation to its opposite, thereby sharpening its disctinctiveness. The participants might think for themselves about the absurdity of reporting all "ugly words" in a detention home, but now the meeting has to proceed.

Passing remarks and insinuations

The examples we have shown here are often aimed at outsiders—such as the clients, other professionals, sometimes obstructing organizations—but there are instances when the meeting participants insert jokes or ironic remarks aimed at each other. At times, such remarks are blatant, as in one of our studies, during the first meetings in a cooperation between border police organizations in the Baltic. The participants are gathered at a castle where conferences are held, and the atmosphere is friendly but serious, and a bit stiff. After the lunch, however, the atmosphere is a bit lighter. When people gather again in the large meeting room, there is a problem with the technical devices that are supposed to run the PowerPoint. The project leader points to his two assistants and says half-flat, half-joking, "Can someone get them out of here? There is no technical equipment that they can't sabotage."

In other cases, one may need quite a long tenure within the organization to detect the irony in such remarks and acquire a refined sensitivity to the local rights and wrongs. One example concerns an episode with Hubert, a psychologist. During a team meeting at a detention home, he presented the case of a young client who needed more therapy. The client would need to deal with his previous crimes, which he did not seem to take responsibility for, no matter how long he and Hubert spent talking about them. The client needs help with "the relational" part, Hubert says to his colleagues during the meeting, arguing that somebody within the detention home with special training in dealing with denying perpetrators should be given this task.

Ylva, the teacher, then responds: "Then it has to be individual talks."

Hubert smiles with a tint of scorn, and replies: "Really?"

This meeting then went on, and other cases were discussed. Hubert's ironic remark, aimed at Ylva's comment, passed quickly. But her *faux pas* or display of relative ignorance—in a detention home, it is self-evident that these kinds of talks should be individual and secluded, and unthinkable that they would occur with an audience—is something the psychologist can point out and subtly question with a minimalist "really?"

Before and after a meeting, there is also room for passing innuendos or remarks, often quite enjoyable and informative for the participants. To arrive on time, sit down, arrange one's meeting props, and chat a little with the others can be an appreciated little ritual, sustaining social bonds and picking up information (Yoerger et al. 2015). During the teachers' meetings that one of us observed, the teachers usually talked with each other in the minutes before the start, exchanging both private and more formal information as well as commenting on daily concerns at work. At one occasion, Ylva, a teacher, sat next to the ethnographer and started to talk about gender studies at detention homes, interviewing him about reports from a gender perspective. She is interested, she says, because "some guys" during her lessons seem to have a very stereotypical view on masculinity and femininity. This is true also when it comes to staff, she says with an insinuating tone. Among the detained young people, some staff have reacted negatively towards such simple stuff as a male client's having a pink notebook, calling it "gay."

> Ylva goes on complaining about the lack of gender diversity tolerance at the detention home and mentions that some guys cultivate "a holy image of the mum." "The mother is a figure one definitely cannot joke about," Ylva says. She smiles, but she then purses her lips a bit. (…) Ylva also says that young girls actually are more violent than the guys, contrary to what you expect. Later on, when the meeting has started, other staff members mention that girls are frequently actors in the statistics on violence at detention homes, and then Ylva looks at me [the fieldworker] and exchanges a glance, as if saying, "Well, what did I tell you?"

Along these lines, informal remarks before a meeting can subtly be drawn upon during the meeting and be incorporated into an argument retrospectively. Ylva exchanges a glance with the fieldworker and reconnects to her pre-meeting remarks on gender during the meeting, thereby infusing some energy into the gathering. She receives some confirmation of her gender perspective—sustaining her performance as informed gender analyst—and she further substantiates her view on violent girls. The exchanged glance symbolizes that there is a discursive line being created that links the informal and slightly biting comments before the meeting with the much more formal and disciplined ones during it.

Other remarks before meetings in our data concern the meeting form as such. Participants, for instance, joke about their need for coffee, their habits of taking the same seat over and over, or their spatial positioning near the exit so that they can leave if the meeting turns too boring. There is often quite a joyful atmosphere in the minutes before a meeting, a relaxed and sometimes slightly teasing or playful feeling among the people, subsequently transformed into formalities when the chairperson starts. The note below refers to the minutes before the teachers' meeting at a detention home:

> Roger jokingly comments on my [the fieldworker's] papers on the table, that they are quite copious. I have brought a thick report on detention homes to read and a notebook, so I really have a pile of paper in front of me. I glance at his place and he also has brought some papers and a notebook. "You need something," Roger says, implying that you cannot participate in these meetings without having something on the table in front of you. Roger sometimes draws pictures during the meetings, for instance. He smiles and looks a little shrewd. "Good, everybody's here then," says Sam, today's chairman. "Somebody has something?"

To "have something" in this context means to have some issues to raise during the meeting, apart from those listed on the agenda. So when Sam says, "everybody's here ..." and asks if somebody "has" something, that is his way of starting the meeting and structuring the discussions. The meeting frame is established, and Roger and the others orient themselves to Sam and the formalities. Just before the meeting, though, there is room for distancing oneself from this frame a bit, and the frame in itself allows it. It is fun to drift back and forth in relation to this form, and it gives energy to the gathering.

Conclusion

By the help of various situations and settings in our studies, we have tried to show how meetings turn seductive in today's administration society. Meetings may obviously harbor attraction in many ways, but this chapter is devoted to an analysis of the forms of interaction we find in ordinary, non-dramatic workplace gatherings. Meetings pull their participants together into shared engagement and effervescence by recurring alterations between formalities and informalities—the one side stimulates the other—so that members of organizations become attracted to meetings, even though they also view meetings as tedious and boring, unnecessarily long, and too frequent.

There is "action" going on during meetings, sometimes in subtle forms, but still: in-house joking and charming identity formations do take place next to dry agendas and stiff meeting personas. The pendulum movement between what organizational members define as formal and what they define as informal is what we would like to point out as the *Eigendynamik*, in Georg Simmel's sense. As researchers, we should not gloss over the details and subtleties of today's long series of meetings and see them merely as a repeated form of social gathering. Rather, we should attend to how members accomplish their movements in and out of this form, artfully loosening it up a bit just to resettle it again, and how this movement contributes to the pull. Meetings express authority, hierarchy, power, and formality, but as people accomplish them, a lot of other things are happening, too. In the next chapter, we look at some other tactics that participants employ to tolerate and even show oblique resistance to meetings that they perceive as boring or not meaningful.

Notes

1 The Swedish daily *Svenska Dagbladet Näringsliv* (2012-12-11) https://www.svd.se/svenska-chefer-halften-av-alla-moten-meningslosa.
2 Researchers have suggested alternatives to the rationalistic model such as Schwartzman's (1989) discussion of meetings as sense-making events; Peck's and colleagues' (2004) discussion of meetings as modern rituals; Boden's (1994) view that meetings are occasions where members produce and reproduce the vision and mission of their organization. Furthermore, Hall and colleagues (2019) suggest a variety of alternatives to the explicit purpose with a meeting: meetings as ways for organizations to organize themselves, meetings as an opportunity to clarify hierarchies, positions among organizations and in between them, and for structuring everyday working life and reality-maintenance among its members.
3 In Kunda's ethnography of engineering culture in a large cooperation, we also see such patterns (2016:131–133), as well as in Bargiela's and Harris's (1997:208–209)) qualitative studies of one British and one Italian company.
4 Rogerson-Revell (2007) has shown how shifts in style between formality and informality are a common feature of business meetings where humor can be used strategically, which facilitate collaboration and inclusion, but also collusion and exclusion.
5 On the concept frame, see Goffman (1974).
6 The type of meeting and whether participants know each other seem to be important for how and when seriousness gives way to play. At the company he studied, Kunda (2006:153–154) reports that it was more common in "work group meetings" that participants interweaved jokes and banter more often in their formal discussions than in other types of meetings (monthly meetings, staff meetings, project meetings, etc.). In work group meetings, people were familiar with each other, but were pressured to "show off," while at the same time they made extensive efforts to suspend and defuse conflict in order to maintain future working relationships. These meetings were characterized by ambiguity, a shared ironic stance and frequent time-outs.

4 Sneaky work and *aways*

In the last chapter, we analyzed tactics related to jocularity in meetings, so let us recall here that meetings are more often commented on in critical ways than they are depicted as fun and appealing. Researchers point to increased administration, and members of organizations grumble over tiring and boring hours in meeting rooms. Complaints about meetings are recurrent in both studies and everyday talk, particularly regarding their frequency, emptiness, and forced attendance, taking time from what employees consider to be their core tasks. Boredom is visible not only in accounts of meetings but also in satirical images (see Image 4.1).

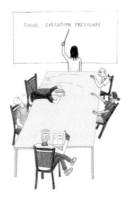

Image 4.1 One of many satirical images delivered in the form of a cartoon.
Source: Image by Axel Åkerström.

Similar cartoons can be found in abundance on the Internet, forming a globalized critique against today's formal meetings, contrasting the meeting organizer's expectations of involvement. Indeed, it is even possible for entrepreneurs to make a business of this culturally accepted image of meetings, as illustrated for instance by the cartoon database and gift shop "Cartoonstock.com," who have a special section for "boring meetings." Here the visitor can choose among 32 boring-meeting cartoons and decide whether to have it printed on a t-shirt or a coffee mug.[1]

DOI: 10.4324/9781003108436-4

We find plenty of retold experiences of boredom in our data, but also observations that may indicate boredom. In the teachers' meeting at the detention home, we found no trace of direct resistance to the meetings as such, but rather micro-practices marking distance and a minimized level of involvement. Participants could yawn, scribble, check their phones, and—as it seemed—daydream with an absent look on their faces as the chair or others talked and showed PowerPoint images. However, attendees did not explicitly oppose the form of gathering nor openly attack it. Various forms of mental removal, though, were evident, occasionally defining the meeting as boring and evidencing an attempt to manage or conquer that feeling with the help of various tactics.

In this chapter, we focus on these tactics. The social control of meetings consists of a moral demand for involvement—participants are supposed to be engaged in and commit themselves to the issues on the agenda—but in practice, actors time and again also distance themselves and temporarily engage in side-involvements or *aways*. There is an observable pendulum movement between involvement and disinvolvement, between control and escape-the-control, and this movement also underlies the *Eigendynamik* of today's meeting society at large. A meeting is an event meant for important things to be discussed and decided, but it also is an event for partly hidden relaxation, daydreaming, sneaky work, and secret islands of relative freedom.

Not passively surrendering

"These meetings," a colleague once said, "are the only occasions I have when I don't feel stressed out." No emails, no pressure to finish any project, submit any text, fulfill others' expectations—the colleague found scheduled meetings to be a safe haven for her, in a period with heavy workload.

(fieldnotes from academia)

Not feeling "stressed out" at meetings, as this academic colleague formulated it, might be interpreted as a relaxing boredom. To find support for our more active interpretation of boredom during meetings—an emotion not necessarily leading to passivity—we turn to Jack Barbalet, who compares it with *ennui* and argues that boredom is slightly different. It is a feeling that expresses "a dissatisfaction with the lack of interest in an activity or condition," but:

Boredom, in its irritability and restlessness (conditions not present in ennui), is not a feeling of acceptance of or resignation toward a state of indifference, as ennui is. Boredom, therefore, is not a passive surrender to those conditions that provoke it.

(Barbalet 1999:634)

At the same time, boredom in meetings is the result of experienced immobility and apathy, and many meetings appear to really cultivate such emotional states. The meeting form guarantees predictability and a sense of stability, but the result might as well be considered too recognizable and repetitious. Boredom is most likely the other side of any kind of emotionally safeguarding standardization. Donna Darden and Alan Marks (1999) describe boredom in terms of a socially disvalued emotion in situations where "the only scripts and props available are too well rehearsed and overly familiar"—a clear contrast to the inserted energizing moments we tried to illustrate in the previous chapter.

> The situation has no apparent future, in sense of anticipation, although it may have a temporal dimension, because time seems to stretch endlessly ahead without a foreseeable denouement.
>
> (Darden and Marks 1999:18)

Swedish author Torgny Lindgren has captured this feeling in a novel called *Övriga frågor* (Swedish for "additions to the agenda"), which revolves around meetings in a small association of the Social Democratic Party in the 1970s. The afternoon meetings were especially depressing, Lindgren writes:

> … when going to them it is still light outside and the world is full of people, then you are enclosed in the meeting, often with a strong sense that time is not moving, neither forwards nor backwards, and when the meeting is over and you get out, it's dark.
>
> (Lindgren, 1973:22, our translation)[2]

The most extreme social-psychological disappearance or *away* during a meeting is probably to fall asleep, as a principal did at times when followed by Harry Wolcott (2003) during his fieldwork. In our data, the instances are more subtle and discreet. The meeting participants can exchange ironic commentaries now and then, abandoning their attention to the meeting for a while. These *aways* are not, as discussed in the previous chapter, a matter of all (or almost all) participants engaging in informal jokes or playfulness as an inserted relaxation of the stiff formalities during a meeting. These are side-involvements by one or a few, hidden from the rest, and giving energy and relieving constraint in a more secluded and individual way.

These *aways* can bracket the chair's or another participant's talk in a manner that reveals that the meeting is subordinated to other activities. But meeting participants also make excuses—in words or gestures—thereby honoring the very ceremonial order of the meeting that is temporarily set aside. Most working life meeting cultures, as the social historian van Vree (1999) has pointed out, have become more and more disciplined. The participant is supposed to listen to the speaker, appear to be interested, and respond in neutral terms, so as not to disturb the ceremonial order of the meeting. To account for one's visible *aways* belongs to the civilized frame of this type of gathering. At the same time, people typically enjoy meetings if they are allowed to co-construct a shared meaning of the event as meaningless, marked with, for instance, exchanged glances or sighs. They can form a temporary community during short intervals and enjoy their unity through making fun of what happens or displaying their moral indignation, and doing so in a way more clearly critical to the administration society than in the examples we showed in the previous chapter.

A niche in the study of side-involvement during meetings should recognize a historical shift where *doodles* seem to become less common because many technical advances such as smartphones, laptops, and iPads have facilitated people's side-involvements. Despite this shift, doodles are still with us as a conventional *away*. Many meeting participants engage in playfully using a pen and paper during meetings, and during our project, we witnessed plenty of examples. One colleague explained to us that drawing random figures and patterns in her notebook was the only way she could stay seemingly alert during faculty meetings, and it worked because nobody really noticed what she was doing. "Scribbling in the margins looks like I am taking notes." Even lawyers in courts, engaged in meetings with a clear involvement and at times high stakes, explain that they scribble in order to stay awake during some period of a trial.[3]

Sneaky work—and private escape routes

People in meetings also engage in "sneaky" or hidden work, that is, doing their *ordinary* work during a meeting, typically through laptops or mobile phones. This work may be done between participants in the same meeting, such as sending emails or text messages to each other, but in the meetings we have studied, sneaky work seems more commonly done by one person for themselves or for external actors. The technique is recurrent: one places oneself to avoid being too visible to the chair—or a speaker in front of an audience—and thereby makes use of cracks or weak spots in the social control. In this way, they are present but partly occupied by something else, appearing to be involved but actually rather absent. To be able to hide such activities depends both on meeting territoriality (Hall, Leppänen, and Åkerström 2019) and the size of the meeting. "Round-table meetings" as well as smaller gatherings increase the potential for mutual monitoring. As illustrated below (Image 4.2), such hidden work need not be done through laptops or mobile phones. It can also be done through ordinary paper books.

Hidden work may also be referred to by participants in talks before or after the meeting and during meeting breaks, so that the significance of the meeting is secretly decreased and more important things are put at the center. Comments on hidden work may be expressed provocatively, as when a scholar complained about an upcoming meeting in his department by

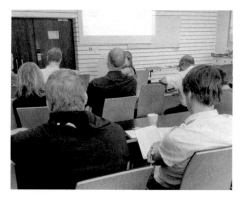

Image 4.2 Participant at a personnel meeting in academia reading Malešević's book *The Sociology of War and Violence* instead of paying attention to the chair or the PowerPoint.
Source: The authors' private photo.

saying, "I plan to write my lecture during the next personnel meeting." But they may also be formulated as confessions:

> During a lunch break at an all-day meeting for personnel at a department, a participant turns to me and one of her colleagues and says in a low voice, while smiling in an apologetic way: "I think I'll try to leave at 15:00. I sneaked in some work during the morning." "So did I," says her colleague, turning to me: "Well these things [discussed during the meeting], we've heard it all before."

Not all such escapes involve work. Games, text messages, private calendars, Facebook posting, and other social media engagement—opportunities are abundant for people in loosely structured or big meetings to escape into side-involvements and get things done in their private lives, too.

Pure "play" may, however, be more morally harmful if discovered, especially if the subjects discussed are framed as having potentially serious consequences for others. This was the case during a public debate in the Norwegian parliament on military defense, involving NATO, when the leader of the political party Venstre, Trine Skei Grande, was discovered playing "Pokémon Go" on her mobile phone.[4] Another politician, the late U.S. senator and Republican presidential candidate John McCain, was discovered playing Internet poker during a Senate hearing on the U.S.–Syria conflict. When publicly exposed, McCain explained ironically:

> As much as I like to always listen in rapt attention constantly to the remarks of my colleagues over a three-and-a-half-hour period, occasionally I get a little bored.[5]

The cases of both Grande and McCain resulted in public shaming, involving not only reports in newspapers but also feedback in publications' online comment sections, such as:

> Love these hacks getting paid on the public's hard-earned dime! Maybe if you're so bored Johnnie [sic] we ought to get a younger, fresher guy who'll pay attention to the taxpayer's needs. Sorry national security is so boring!!![6]

But even less conspicuous and widespread cases may cause embarrassment as meeting participants mutually monitor each other. One meeting participant told us how she started to play a private video of her kids during a particularly dull meeting and did not realize that the sound was on, which was very embarrassing. Another told about watching the presidential debate during a meeting and accidentally putting on the sound—which also was embarrassing and drew many surprised and irritated looks. The same digital equipment and devices that facilitate *aways*, such as laptops, iPads, and smartphones, also facilitate mutual surveillance and embarrassing leakages of side-involvement.

As Goffman (1967/1982:86) noted in writing on deference and demeanor: "Profanations are to be expected, for every religious ceremony creates the possibility of a black mass." There are, however, instances when meeting the demands of the meeting ceremony while perceiving the meeting as boring may be transformed into fun.

The boring qualities and the ceremonial order are exactly the factors that produce humor and irony. Humor inhabits situations and places found in incongruity, in contrasts between the expected and unexpected, in two incompatible views of a scene. The humor often derives its punch from an implicit perspective containing a rational expectation of meetings: a social form that rationally and instrumentally enables and directs collective action to a certain goal. Entire TV comedy series have taken this focus. For example, *The Office* is based on working in a boring office and all the dull things that one has to put up with, countered by infusions of energy through humor, shared practical jokes, and individual *aways*.

The satirical image shown, taken from the Internet, is one such instance. In our data, we have also found such examples in fieldnotes. One illustration was collected during a two-day meeting attended by teachers and researchers at a university in northern Sweden:

> Before the meeting starts, we sit and drink coffee outside. It's sunny and nice, people do not want to leave for the conference room. We decide to wait for the dean and chair to call us. After a while, we see them stand up at a distance and chat with each other but not calling us, one at the table mutters "So, *now* they plan this conference," "Don't be nasty," says another. "Well, let's see if it's more coherent or as meaningless as last year." "You look shocked"—to a new employee, who smiles: "I'm new, don't dare to make comments."

In the large conference room, about 50 people are gathered, and we sit at different tables for four people, all turned towards the front where the dean who chairs the meeting is standing. When she reads the agenda from a PowerPoint slide, I manage to catch a few sarcastic comments. The second item on the agenda says: "Written feedback from last meeting." One of the participants whispers: "Yippee." Then the chair reads aloud from a PowerPoint shown on the screen in front of the room, point by point: it's the agenda for the two upcoming days. Someone close to me [the researcher] points discreetly to the screen and says, "everything is up there, we can read, no one here is blind," meaning "why does she have to read the agenda aloud?"

Later on, in the afternoon, the dean ends a discussion with, "We'll take this issue with us" [in Swedish "vi tar med oss frågan"] when someone writes a note to me, "Typical meeting cliché, but nothing ever happens." Before we leave for group discussions, someone asks, "At what time is the coffee break?" "At 15:00." "I'll set the alarm for that then," and someone else looks around and ask for a member supposed to be in his group. "Where is Anna Bengtsson?" "She's gone home." "Well, that was a smart decision."

All of these comments are ironic and form part of the humorous exchanges—and a mild form of enjoyment in small subgroups of the meeting, sustaining the understanding of a temporary "We."

It is not a matter of more universal and open sharing of such moments described in the previous chapter; the dynamic is different because the meeting is larger and it is more difficult to unite all under a shared purpose. Such subgroups or temporary "We's" are often built on an earlier trusted relationship—people whom one knows and thus are expected to welcome such mutterings and irony. This was the case in this meeting. Moreover, such moments may cement allegiances and harbor narrative possibilities, sometimes also recalling previous moments of fun (Fine and Corte 2017). They work a bit different than the more globally shared humor described in the previous chapter, marking the underlife of the administration society rather than merely pauses from it.

A subversive, less-than-candid little "rebellion" in the margins nonetheless contribute to the reproduction of meeting chains, since no open protest is articulated. Things can go on as usual, and more meetings can be suggested without objections.

Moreover, what may be boring to one person could be fascinating and meaningful to someone else; boredom is not intrinsic to any event or object. Czarniawska-Joerges (1992:33) discusses how shared meaning might not be crucial for collective action, and she gives the following illustration:

My two colleagues went to hear a speech by a well-known businessman. One "participated in a most exciting encounter between the wisdom of practice and curiosity of theory," whereas the other "took part in an extremely boring meeting with an elderly gentleman who told old jokes." They are each, nevertheless, members of the same organization, and what was common for them was that they went to the same room at the same hour, sharing only the idea that their bosses expected it.

What makes for involvement and disinvolvement? In the previous case, it might be the content of the speech or the way it was delivered. But we want to point to a few more sociological points.

The first theme relates to the individual roles of the attendees and what captures their interest as relevant to that role. Often, meetings gather a number of people whose interests are associated with only some or one of the issues on the agenda that will be discussed or decided. A school's economist may be quite inattentive when listening to a new proposal for schedules but wake up when the budget will be discussed. Meetings with broad agendas and many different areas of interests (such as faculty meetings, board meetings, etc.) work differently than the ones with more specific agendas and smaller groups of attendees. If the meeting is large and displays clear hierarchies, in-house jokes or other types of inserted and energizing breaks from the formalities seem less favored than more individual or small-scale *aways*.

Furthermore, there is also a sociological element regarding ascribed roles and division of labor that influences how meetings are experienced differently. Our interviews of chairs in different departments made evident that they differentiated between meetings in which they were the chair and those they had to attend to as ordinary meeting participants. As one informant explained: "When you attend the large faculty meeting where the dean informs all the chairs from different departments, it becomes very much 'informing us', rather boring, that's when you start looking at your emails, and so on." But being chair oneself is involving, it demands orchestrating and directing the meeting, and it demands attention. Moreover, a chair might have a plan of what the meeting is to accomplish. Thus, in interviews, managers explain that when they are chairs, even though they are caught in their meetings, they are usually not bored, in contrast to meetings that they do not chair. Where the individual is situated in the hierarchies that are displayed during a meeting seems to play a role for his or her feelings or boredom.

A second theme concerns both variations of meetings and changing norms in meeting culture about multitasking. When one retired civil servant we interviewed compared his meeting experiences, he emphasized the more common use of laptops and mobile phones during his last working years even in elite, formal meetings. This behavior would have been unthinkable before but had now become perfectly acceptable. Wasson (2006) has studied virtual meetings where people routinely multitask during the meetings. They prefer to stay in their own, individual offices and "attend" meetings virtually for this reason, rather than being present in a conference room.

A third theme concerns handling the boredom of others. Chairs sometimes notice when others are bored. In our interviews with chairs and managers who lead meetings, they talk about noticing when people start nodding, drawing doodles, playing with phones, or looking at their watches. When asked how they respond, a head of a unit at a detention home answers:

> In the afternoon, when you see them sitting like this [the interviewee bends forward, head in his hands, looking down], then you may say: "Well, now we'll take a coffee break."

But one may also use participants' perceived boredom as an excuse to keep meetings as short as possible, as a chair explained: "Don't let them open the window, do not take a coffee break. Such initiatives will make the meeting go on forever."

If meeting participants sometimes have to engage in emotional management to hide being bored, representatives of the meeting industry instead promise "emotional achievements" through an engaging and involving meeting. The ambitions of the burgeoning meeting industry to shape more effective meetings are partly founded on these promises of the meeting designers, facilitators, and consultants to construct an affective atmosphere (Andersson Cederholm 2010) that will ensure creativity, authenticity, and intimacy. In the meeting consultancy business, tips on how to create both more fun, energizing, engaging, and effective meetings are abundant. One example is variations on the notion of "checking in" in meetings, in order to specify the aim and expectations of the meetings. This means that all participants briefly say what they expect from the meeting. This is described as energizing, and a way to create focus and a sense of inclusion. The meeting room as such and the physical environment are also highlighted as important in the consultancy literature. The choice of meeting room should be adapted to the purpose of the meeting, as explained by a meeting consultant who calls himself a "meeting evangelist": "There will be a difference between the energy created in a meeting held under a huge oak-tree a sunny day, compared to the meeting held in a soul-less conference room with stripped white walls."[7] Furthermore, meeting consultancy magazines often focus on the importance of bodily functions, with tips on the best meeting food and drink to stay alert and active, as well as various analyses of bodily movements during meetings. To "walk and talk" is promoted as a new meeting form.[8]

To have fun in meetings and consequently fighting boredom and the associated *aways* are the goal for the meeting industry, ultimately sharpening a smart version of social control at the workplaces. "Fun," as Fine and Corte (2017:68) write, "is not merely pleasurable action but action that produces social cohesion, in contrast to alienating forces of routine and coercion."

Conclusion

In this chapter, we have analyzed the underlife of today's meeting culture within the organizations we include in our studies and how it paradoxically sustains the production of endless chains of meetings. Meeting participants may daydream and doodle, engage in gaming or sneaky work coupled with private digital errands, or in other ways escape temporarily through discreet use of smartphones and laptops (and the like), but while doing so, they also pay silent respect to the formalities taking place on stage. As members of various formal gatherings develop and employ tactics to survive boredom and rigidity, they simultaneously contribute to stability.

Our data are full of tactical responses and maneuvers that circumvent some of the administrative control of today's meeting culture, whereas direct and open resistance to "yet another meeting" (or a prolonged one) is much rarer. *Aways* and side-involvements, we argue, are part and parcel of what is going on: temporary escapes and discreet pauses that help sustain the apparatus.

We have also tried to show how a standardized, overly familiar, and well-rehearsed working format seems to invite rather than dismiss *aways* and side-involvements, which is probably what the meeting industry and its consultants try to fight (Andersson Cederholm 2010; Andersson Cederholm and Hall 2019). They want innovation: new forms of meetings, engaging props, and surprising events which, if efficient, would put an end to the underlife creativity.

Most likely, though, the latter will not happen. In our data, members find their ways whether managers try out innovative meeting forms or not. It is not only technological development that allows us to try multitasking more and more but also our extensive and continuous training as meeting participants.

In the next chapter, we look at how meeting participants and organizers also use the "magic of documentation" to perpetuate the eternal meeting, generating tangible deliverables to create an illusion of the concrete from the abstract.

Notes

1 https://www.cartoonstock.com/directory/b/boring_meetings.asp. Retrieved 14/11/2020.
2 In original: "Det är också beklämmande med dessa eftermiddagsmöten: när man går dit är det ännu ljust i världen och fullt av medmänniskor, sedan sitter man innesluten i mötet, ofta med en stark känsla av att tiden inte rör sig, varken framåt eller bakåt, och när mötet är över och man kommer ut är det mörkt" (Lindgren 1973:22).
3 Personal communication with Lisa Flower who examines emotional themes pertaining to being a lawyer (Flower, 2019).
4 https://www.dagensps.se/foretagare/opinion/partiledare-jagar-pokemon-go-pa-jobbet/. Retrieved 07/02/2021.

5 https://www.washingtonpost.com/news/post-politics/wp/2013/09/04/mccain-on-smartphone-poker-i-get-a-little-bored/#comments. Retrieved 07/02/2021.
6 The comments section of this article is no longer accessible.
7 https://www.foretagande.se/personal/moten-med-energi. Retrieved 07/02/2021.
8 https://hbr.org/2015/08/how-to-do-walking-meetings-right. Retrieved 07/02/2021.

5 A spark of magic

In the preceding chapter, we examined how meeting participants navigate meeting boredom through the creation of hidden individual or subgroup distractions. They use sleight of hand to disguise their lack of interest in the proceedings. In this chapter, we look at a different kind of illusion: the use of documents to create in an almost magical way a concrete reality from difficult-to-quantify abstractions.

Human services work carried out in democratic societies takes place as much in a legal context as an institutional one, and documentation is vital for running, representing, justifying, and accounting for such work. Meticulous documentation may operate as a formal memory bank for what is considered to have happened and what conclusions to draw for future recommendations. Patient and client rights are supposed to be acknowledged and protected, and staff is accountable for the care provided or not provided. Still, honored but abstract ideas such as "care," "collaboration," "prevention," and "quality" are not easy to capture. For this reason, among others, documents have a prominent position in human services work: records, guidelines, and plans tend to manifest, encapsulate, and pinpoint elusive qualities in written forms (Prior 2003).

Documentation in human services organizations represents the ability to turn quite diffuse activities and responsibilities into things (e.g., plans, agreements, records), and these things (documents) attain rather vital properties, sometimes even magical ones, as we will argue in this chapter. For example, research on complaints in elder care has shown that although the complaint itself typically is about lack of care, the regulatory authority responding to it focuses on deficiencies *in the very documentation* (Kjellberg 2019). If the nursing home can present the requested plans and documents, they are likely to be assessed as a respected establishment that provides "quality care." If they cannot do so, they run the risk of a lower score in quality measurements. To "have" a care plan in its documentary form equates to "having" quality (Jacobsson and Martinell Barfoed 2019).

In this way, a care plan turns into a reified proof of quality. When quality is manifested in certain kinds of documents, these particular documents tend to attain powerful properties. Correctly filled out care plans can be the

DOI: 10.4324/9781003108436-5

key to approval from the authorities who present rankings of nursing homes, youth care facilities, health care, and more. An Equal Treatment Plan—a plan against discrimination and offensive treatment—can contribute to high scores in external quality measurements, as would the procedure of merely *providing* the Annual Service User Questionnaire (in order to get feedback from service users), not necessarily its results. The documents themselves are used as evidence of quality (or care, collaboration, prevention, etc.) in various rankings, for example of a nursing home, regardless of, or disconnected from, the experiences that staff and clients gain (cf. Carlstedt and Jacobsson 2017). Ultimately, such *documentary magic* can be vital to the survival and prosperity of a human services organization—or any organization really—when rankings direct clients and patients or customers to "the best" places and to methods "that work."

It is difficult to underestimate the importance of the written word when authority decisions are to be exercised. Let us give another example. The tragic death of Palestinian 8-year-old Yara seeking refuge in Sweden in 2015 was much debated and generated massive media coverage nationally and to a lesser extent internationally.[1] The social services had decided that Yara should stay with her uncle and his wife and did not react until it was too late to report against the couple concerning their serious neglect and maltreatment of Yara. She was mistreated and beaten, and investigations after her death suggested that Yara had endured physical abuse for some time. While the legal pursuit of Yara's murderers was ongoing, a bureaucratic chase also took place. A number of accusations were made in the media against the authorities who were portrayed as responsible for the girl's fate: the social services, the police department, and the school. The principal had not made a formal report when he contacted the social services to inquire about the girl's home situation. A police officer sent a fax with the heading "Info about possible 'Maladjustment' in the home" to the social services offices, which were closed for Easter. There the fax was left for a week because the case worker was on vacation for a couple more days. Even when the fax was received, the worker did not take action because the heading and the use of fax as a means of communication were not perceived to signal an alarming situation. In short, one missing formal report, one unread fax, and the word choice in a heading: three flawed administrative routines that in news headlines were pointed out as factors opening the way to Yara's being killed a few days later. In the bureaucratic chase, causes of tragic events such as Yara's death are primarily sought in potentially defective routines. These routines are often synonymous with documentary routines because what remains from a past event of human services provision is the paperwork (Jacobsson and Martinell Barfoed 2019).

The paperwork (or requested paperwork) in these examples related above, from elder care and social services child care, are instances of legitimation, self-justification, or audit trails. Actions taken or not taken can be legitimized and justified with the proper bureaucratic formula, and the produced documents can be traced for audit in retrospect.

We want to draw attention to the magical qualities of such documentary practices: how they are socially invoked and accomplished. We refer to a kind of "sympathetic magic" in the sense of "like produces like," as anthropologist Marcel Mauss (2001) discussed. For example, in the settings that anthropologists studied at the time of Mauss's work, the rainmaker was believed to entice real clouds and rain by mimicking heavy rainfall in dances and simulating dark clouds with the burning of fresh branches. The purpose with magic, in this respect, is to produce concrete and actual results. Translated to a bureaucratic environment: *order is a desirable result.* If the paperwork is in order, then the activities, procedures, and conducts in an organization are believed to actually be in order, or at least the probability of their being so is increased. When order is believed to produce order, disorder is believed to produce disorder. In Yara's case, the failure in administrative routines "produced" the failure to care for a child, as the members of the involved bureaucracies defined it. In the case of the nursing home, a care plan "produced" care. According to this somewhat magical logic, paperwork represents and reconstructs what is actually done and accomplished in the organization.

This chapter will illustrate such "magical properties" of documents with the help of two cases. First, we discuss how *preventive social work* is accomplished by being captured in numbers on paper. Second, we turn to how *collaboration* may be manifested in documentary form, documents that work as a token of collaboration between authorities. Both cases involve reification processes (Berger and Luckmann 1967), where documents eventually are made into objective artifacts that supposedly represent the state of being and somehow seem to be detached from the humans who initially produced them. We are particularly interested in how such reification processes grant considerable power to documents and thereby fuel the *Eigendynamik* of today's administration society.

Preventive social work in figures

Political and economic development in the area of human services work tends to favor rampant quantification. Measures of various kinds (e.g., standards, statistics, indicators) have come to dominate human services to such an extent that contemporary public management is described as "governing by numbers" (Shore and Wright 2015). For example, measurement cultures stand out in social work where the quantifiable has superior value, directing both management and staff towards measuring social work (Hjärpe 2020). The notion that "only what's counted counts" leads to inventive procedures among staff to count and document even when doing so is not stipulated by rules or conventions. The aim of this "extra documentation" is to prove that work has been carried out, making work processes or work results visible to decision makers up the hierarchical ladder and presenting the employees as competent and busy.

This proxy of proof was the case in our material in one of the few divisions at the social services where documentation is meant to be kept to a minimum—fieldwork among young people in the streets. Here, at the division "Social workers for youth," fieldworkers started to produce statistics themselves. The manager of the division initiated this practice to make visible that preventive social work actually took place in the city, a practice that was undetectable without the regular currency of documents (such as countable plans and treatment enrollments). In fear of cutbacks, the manager wanted to make sure the fieldworkers' workload was measured and visualized. The self-initiated statistics served the purpose of speaking the predominant quantified authority language, in which numbers convey objectivity and power (Best 2012).

Preventive social work is not easily defined. Fieldworkers "hang around," making themselves available to young people sometimes just by being there and sometimes as an active conversational partner. The working method is characterized by rather mundane practices. But with this initiative on the part of the manager, the details in preventive work had to be spelled out: everything named, specified, and classified to make counting possible (Bowker and Star 1999). The fieldworkers were instructed to log every conversation they had with young people during their shift, classify the type of conversation, and specify the topic. The rather intricate documentary process involved four steps.

Step 1

First, at the site, fieldworkers completed a pre-printed small template of the size 10 × 15 cm (Image 5.1). They were not allowed to keep records with names and personal details, and the youngsters they approached (or were approached by) are legally not to be seen as clients. The loggings were thus made for purely statistical reasons, gathering information on the number of youths, their gender and age, and whether they were known beforehand to the social services, suspected to lead "a criminal lifestyle," or at risk of doing so.

Furthermore, the type of conversation was logged according to three broad categories: "encouraging," "supportive," or "advice-giving."[2] Each category was classified into around 15 conversational topics for the fieldworker to choose from (e.g., work, school, sexuality, alcohol). Below is an example of a completed template, with the following information: fieldworkers have had an "encouraging" conversation with four "new" boys (i.e., unknown to the social services), ages 12–17, and it is unclear if they lead a criminal lifestyle or are at risk of doing so. The conversation took place at 10 minutes past midnight in "OPS" (short for Olof Palme Square). They talked about leisure time and the social services. In the lower-right corner, the fieldworker has jotted "bus t," meaning that she handed out bus tickets to the boys for the journey home. It also says that the boys would like to have a more fun carnival next year (this was during the city's annual carnival) and that they think the fieldworker division "is good."

Fieldnotes and statistics   08.10 OPS

Time and place : _____

Youths 12–17 years	Total	New	At risk	Criminal lifestyle	No risk	Don't know
						4
Boys	4	4				
Girls						

Young adults 18–21 years	Total	New	At risk	Criminal lifestyle	No risk	Don't know
Boys						
Girls						

Type of talk or intervention

Encouraging No. 4	Supportive No.	Advice-giving No.
Work	Living	Living
School	Work	Work
Future	School	School
Relations	Mental health	Relations
Sex/sexuality	Relations	Sex/sexuality
Leisure time 4	Sex/sexuality	Leisure time
Social services 4	Leisure time	Victim of crime
Police	Victim of crime	Alcohol
Drugs	Alcohol	Narcotics
Family	Narcotics	Criminality
Society/politics	Criminality	Family
O. relationship	Family	Social services
O. safekeeping	Social services	Police
Other	Police	Other
	Other	

Assessment talk	
Worry talk	
Handed over to authority	
Helped youth to get home	

Bus t. Want more for carnaval next year. Think S4Y is good.

Image 5.1 Step 1: Youth fieldworker's template after logging a conversation with four boys in a square around midnight. The worker categorized the conversation as "encouraging" (not "supportive" or "advice-giving") on the topics "leisure time" and "the social services." The purpose with documenting each contact with young people thoroughly is to gather material for statistical compilation of the city's preventive social work. The template is reconstructed for reasons of translation and anonymity.

The templates were filled out after a conversation had taken place and out of sight of the youths themselves. The fieldworkers made extensive efforts to keep their recordings hidden from all young people in the streets according to ideas that taking notes would spoil trust and make the youth less keen to talk to them. In addition to the templates, workers were equipped with a tally counter to "click" on every occasion of the slightest contact with a young person. They were told to click even when just saying "hi" to someone, to "get the statistics up."

Step 2

The second step in documenting the work shift took place at the office, just before the fieldworker finished the shift. Now, the numbers and crosses on the templates (and the results from the tally counter) were transferred digitally to an Excel sheet (Image 5.2).

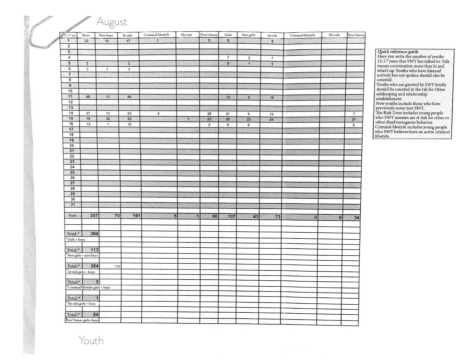

August / Youth

12–17 yrs	Boys	New boys	At risk	Criminal lifestyle	No risk	Don't know	Girls	New girls	At risk	Criminal lifestyle	No risk	Don't know
1	23	10	17	1			5	6	6			
2												
3												
4							7	2	7			
5	3		3				5	1	5			
6	3	1	3									
7												
8												
9												
10												
11	40	13	40				12	2	12			
12												
13												
14	97	13	65	4			28	21	9	14		7
15	79	32	63		1		25	60	23	29		21
16	12	1	10				2	6	6			6
17												
18												
19												
20												
21												
22												
23												
24												
25												
26												
27												
28												
29												
30												
31												
Sum	257	70	191	5	1	60	107	43	73	0	0	34

Total:*	364		*Girls + boys
Total:*	113		*New girls + new boys
Total:*	264	73%	*At risk girls + boys
Total:*	5		*Criminal lifestyle girls + boys
Total:*	1		*No risk girls + boys
Total:*	94		*Don't know girls + boys

Quick reference guide
Here you write the number of youths 12–17 years that SWY has talked to. Talk means conversation more than hi and what's up. Youths who have listened actively but not spoken should also be counted.
Youths who are greeted by SWY briefly should be counted in the tab for Other safekeeping and relationship establishment.
New youths include those who have previously never met SWY.
The Risk Zone includes young people who SWY assesses are at risk for crime or other disadvantageous behavior.
Criminal lifestyle includes young people who SWY believes have an active criminal lifestyle.

Image 5.2 Step 2: Before finishing a shift, fieldworkers were obliged to transfer the figures on their handwritten templates into an Excel sheet. Above is a compilation of fieldworker templates collected during one month, serving as a basis for statistical presentations made by the division manager. The Excel sheet is reconstructed for reasons of translation and anonymity.

Quantification of professional assessments generate considerable work, not the least to establish definitions of what the numbers stand for (Espeland and Stevens, 2008), and manuals and guidelines serve to guarantee a shared practice among professionals. This also is the case here: In addition to the tables, a quick reference guide explains how fieldworkers are supposed to count the youth: What does "talk" mean? More than just "Hi" and "What's up?" What if the kids don't say anything? Where should the very brief greetings be filed? An extract from the Excel sheet:

Quick-reference guide
Here you write the number of youth 12–17 years with whom SWY [Social Workers for Youth] has talked. Talk means conversation more than "Hi" and "What's up?" Youth who have listened actively but did not speak should also be counted.
Youth who are greeted by SWY briefly should be counted in the tab for Other safekeeping and relationship establishment. /---/

The quick-reference guide also provides definitions of who is to be considered "new" and who is in a "risk zone" or leads a "criminal lifestyle":

> New youth include those who have previously never met SWY.
> The risk zone includes young people whom SWY assesses are at risk for crime or other disadvantageous behavior.
> Criminal lifestyle includes young people whom SWY believes have an active criminal lifestyle.

Still, these guidelines are no more precise than an appeal to the fieldworkers' assessments and beliefs. Vagueness and uncertainty vanish as soon as the Excel sheet is completed and transformed into figures. For example, we can see that in August, the fieldworkers talked to 70 "new boys" and 43 "new girls." Out of all 364 young people (not counting the new girls and boys), 73% were classified as at risk. One boy was clearly not at risk, whereas five boys led a criminal lifestyle. Uncertainty can also be quantified: In 94 cases, the fieldworkers chose to tick "don't know."

Other Excel sheets were even more divided and detailed. During a given time period, they specify what kind of conversation was held, with how many boys and girls, and what the topic of the conversation was. By the end of the month, all numbers were compiled for statistical calculation and presentation by the division manager.

Step 3

The third step consists of so-called field notes in a diary (Image 5.3). After the numbers are fed into the Excel sheet, less formalized notes are written, printed, and put in a file before the fieldworkers head home after a completed shift. The notes serve the purpose of allowing the staff to keep up with what has happened and are saved for 12 months. Fieldworkers are told to write something about every conversation they have during a night, and the diary notes have to add up to match the Excel statistics. This request was often hard to fulfill, says one of the fieldworkers, and caused a lot of headache and confusion in the effort to get both documents to match each other.

The diary shows the documentary orientation to the legally defined non-documentary character of fieldwork. Because fieldworkers are engaged in preventive work and all contacts with young people are voluntary, they are not allowed to document by name and individual personal numbers. Like the common routines of keeping a logbook at, for example, detention homes or nursing homes, the field notes are said to give the next shift of fieldworkers an idea of what happened on earlier shifts. Unlike institutions with identifiable clients, patients, or guests, the fieldworkers walk the city streets, meeting young people at random. Only once in a while do they know a youth's name, and it is not certain that the same youth will show up next week.

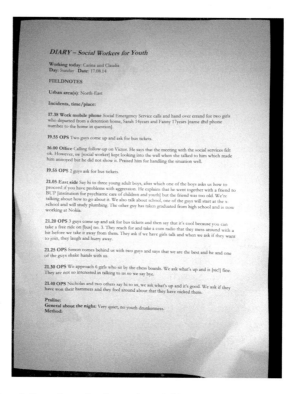

Image 5.3 Step 3: Page from the diary where fieldworkers note what happened during their shift in a more narrative form, as opposed to the figures in previous steps. This diary page has been reconstructed with pseudonyms and to remove identifying information for the purpose of translation and anonymity.

Some comments seem relevant for passing on information, such as the note about two teenage girls who have departed from a detention home without permission. Sometimes a few well-known youths are observed frequently during a period of time and may be named by nicknames or first names, which makes it possible to keep track of their whereabouts. But why do fieldworkers take notes like, "Two guys approach and ask for bus tickets," and "We approach 6 girls who sit by the chess boards. We ask what's up and is [sic!] fine. They are not so interested in talking to us so we say bye"? The answer to the meticulous note-taking is that, first of all, the documentary approach is predominant in all human services work, and logbook notes often operate as an organizing principle when staff report to the next shift. Second, the diary or other logbooks give an opportunity to present this work in detail and give evidence of actual work performed. Third, in this particular case, fieldworkers were told to log "every conversation" to make the diary match the statistics. The different kinds of documents used in this four-step procedure were entangled with each other and produced with the next step in mind.

Step 4

The fourth and final step in making the workload visible was solely in the hands of the division manager, who in this case spent one day per week compiling the material generated in the previous three steps. Based on the statistics, she produced bar graphs and diagrams for every month, printed on thick, heavyweight A3 paper, and nailed to a display board at the office (Image 5.4).

We know the categories and classifications from the template in the first step, which are now shown in the distribution of different kinds of talks the fieldworkers have had with young people and their identification of how many

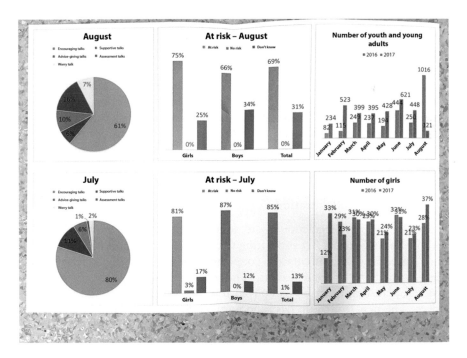

Image 5.4 Step 4: Bars, figures, and diagrams made by the division manager, based on the information in the fieldworkers' templates. Printed on a heavyweight paper, size A3. Its significance is indicated by the fact that it is nailed to a display board at the office. The figures and posters are used to present a busy social services division and legitimize its very existence. The text is translated.

kids were at risk or not. We learn that youth walking the streets at night seldom can be classified as "no risk," at least not with certainty. The numbers of youth and young adults are compared with those of the previous year, giving a clear picture of a steady rise in numbers (apart from August, which was explained by a sudden crisis in the city when all fieldworkers were reallocated to other work tasks). One square of the displayed material is devoted to depicting the proportion of girls with whom the fieldworkers talked. Boys were more likely to approach fieldworkers for a chat, so one goal was to expand the conversations with girls. Taken together, the graphs not only show a busy fieldworker group but also visualize that the great majority of young people out there are at risk, their numbers rising from one year to another, with young girls making up a fairly large proportion of them.

From just this brief look at the material, it is not difficult to detect several errors and mistakes in the procedure of gathering and presenting statistical data. The whole project seems somewhat amateurish. Just to mention but a few examples: The boy who was not at risk in the Excel sheet is not represented in the poster diagrams, the numbers don't always add up (for example, 101% girls and 99% boys), and the label "number of girls" is misleading because the graph actually depicts the proportion of girls. But these flaws are not important. The colorful posters serve as precisely the kind of statistical ammunition a manager needs when requesting more resources or when already allocated resources are questioned (Hjärpe 2020). As such, they may work in magical ways, in line with Mauss' (2001) reasonings. They encapsulate fieldworkers' invisible working methods and clearly visualize efforts that otherwise seem to evaporate in an organization where documentation and measurements are standard procedure. With these graphs and figures, voilà! Here you have it—preventive social work transformed into hard facts. Order in numbers and diagrams equals the keeping of order in the street.

Inscriptions of collaboration

A decade ago, new regulations were added to the Swedish Health Care Act and the Social Services Act stipulating that municipalities and county councils must enter into agreements on cooperation regarding people with service needs from both of these sectors. The agreement is materialized in an individual plan that must be completed together with patients and (often) relatives. The new legislation has been particularly accentuated through various efforts to regulate and formalize collaboration with the help of education, guidelines, and handbooks. Efforts to standardize collaboration between authorities tie into a general trend in standardizing many aspects of human services work (Timmermans and Epstein 2010; White, Hall, and Peckover 2009), and "collaboration" is described as a self-evidently successful working method often enough that it has become a policy instrument in itself (Lascoumes and Le Gales 2007).

Swedish research on collaboration is typically normative in relating topics such as how obstacles for collaboration can be removed and the importance of consensus between different professional groups when collaborating (e.g., Nordström 2016; Widmark 2015). Collaboration has seldom been examined as a phenomenon per se in Swedish research (but see, for example, Basic 2018).

Following the shared idea of collaborative hardships, Swedish authorities launched an individual treatment plan as a solution. The related document is called a SIP, a Coordinated Individual Plan,[3] in which the collaboration among different care providers can be manifested. In practice, it means that the involved agencies meet to draw up a plan for the client or patient, stating "who does what and when." There is not a fixed template for the SIP, but all human services or health organizations are constructing one for their own practical purposes. Below is an example of a fairly straightforward SIP form (Image 5.5), but gradually over time, various versions of the SIP form have become more detailed with more subheadings and pages.

A SIP is presented as a tool for providing good care, tailored to the individual client's needs. In recent years, the SIP has been subject to an implementation campaign to bring about its consistent and regular use within all Swedish municipalities and county councils. In meetings and conferences, websites and newsletters, staff have been informed about "SIP—a tool for collaboration." It is a document freighted by great hopes, and at some points, SIP has been characterized as "the reform of the decade!"[4] The launching of the SIP has similarities to the emergence and spreading of what Joel Best (2006) calls *institutional fads*: a problem is defined (clients are "falling between the cracks"), and a solution is presented ("a SIP").

Organizational agreements, individual plans, or official meetings cannot guarantee successful collaboration, which is rather constructed and reconstructed in everyday interactions, as through discursive exchanges, conflicts, joint efforts, and alliance formations (Basic 2018). Like "preventive social work," "collaboration" is accomplished by actors' mundane practices that are hard to specify and pin down. But the SIP offers an opportunity for organizations and professionals to manifest collaboration in black and white. As with the acceptance of well-executed documents as faithful proxies for quality in elder care, documented collaboration becomes proof of "actual" collaboration in assessments of a unit's "outputs" and is equated with quality care. But some doctors, nurses, and social workers view SIP as yet another administrative burden and say they develop ways to navigate around the paperwork by not calling a collaboration meeting a "SIP meeting" (Rönnqvist 2019). Other methods are to circumvent the manual for conducting a SIP meeting by rationalizing away certain elements, sometimes even the physical meeting with the patient or client (Rönnqvist 2019), which was the original purpose for the introduction of the SIP.

The document itself has become particularly important for its function as a token of quality, which is why managers forcefully push for "doing a SIP"

Date:_____

Name/social security number: _____ _____

COORDINATED INDIVIDUAL PLAN

Plan for personal development

Participants:_____
_____
_____
_____ _____

Long term personal goal:

_____

Goals I want to achieve in the next few months:

_____
_____
_____
_____

The child perspective:

_____

_____

What's it like now?

_____

_____

Who do what and when?

_____

_____

_____

Date for Evaluation: _____

Coordinator for this plan is: _____

Image 5.5 An example of a rather plain SIP form, only one page long. Gradually over time, other SIP forms in various local settings have been more elaborated and often contain more pages and subheadings (this SIP form is reconstructed for reasons of anonymity and translation).

in both primary care and the social services. Managers call for a general increase in the quantity of completed SIPs, along with setting standard values for how many SIPs are expected for a given population. At one meeting with the social services and elementary school principals, for example, a counselor drew attention to the fact that they had carried out far too few SIPs in the region. In an upset tone of voice, she explained: "For a hundred children, there should be one SIP. This means between five to seven SIPs per school!" These were numbers that the municipality in question were far from reaching.

Within primary care, economic incentives from central authorities are linked to the completion of a SIP, in which one SIP equals 3000 Swedish kronor (ca. 300 Euros) allocated to the primary care unit where the SIP is completed. One division manager in our material tells about how they had managed to attract 1.3 million Swedish kronor in what she called "ice-cream money", (in Swedish: *glasspengar*) that is, extra money for carrying out SIPs and home visits, among other things. "The most important thing," she says, "is of course that it generates quality for the patient, but also three thousand kronor, and five production pins." The manager acknowledges the extra administrative burden for doctors and nurses, but suggests that the staff turn it into something positive instead. She exemplifies: "Like the other day, Elsa [a doctor] said to me: 'Ka-ching! Today I've made 6000!' I guess that was two SIPs in a day."

When the SIP was launched as "a tool for collaboration" in a campaign-like manner (see Chapter 6), it seemed inevitable that the document itself and its administrative process would attract much attention. Questions regarding the importance of "drawing up a SIP," when it should be done, and how it should be done tend to overshadow how to achieve the collaboration in practice. In the process, focus shifts from actual collaboration to procedural and technical concerns around the form and its associated meetings, which reproduces and strengthens the administration society.

Handbooks provide checklists for the participants on how to prepare for a SIP meeting, including how to inform the individual patient and practical matters such as booking a meeting room. Other topics cover how to structure a meeting and how to talk to a different occupational group from one's own. There are also separate manuals for the digital handling of the SIP system. During this "administrative evolution," the completion of a SIP document has become collaboration in itself and now "quality" refers to "doing a SIP with quality." For example, the Swedish Association of Local Authorities and Regions (SALAR) created a slideshow entitled "Good SIP quality" that consists of 22 slides discussing how the SIP *process* should be carried out. There is no mention of what collaboration means in terms of specific working tasks except that all participants have to "believe in collaboration" to succeed.

Conclusion

Human services work is often messy and sometimes unpredictable. Client situations and need for help are not always straightforward and can require sensitivity and an approach that considers uniqueness or ambiguity. In addition, the work itself may be complicated. Rules and regulations must be followed, different professions and authorities are supposed to collaborate, and certain practical procedures and routines should be honored.

Our research has shown that such intricate work tasks are disentangled and seemingly diminished or displaced when they are instead portrayed as unequivocal and clear-cut with the help of standardized documents, as in the case of the youth fieldworkers and the four-step process we describe in this chapter. Moreover, these documents seem to possess magic-like properties so that the document in itself manifests the sought-after qualities that are the goal, as in our example from elder care for quality assurance and with the SIP as a proxy for functional collaboration. Despite the illusory quality of such documents, here we also have exemplified with preventive social work and collaboration that such practices, when reified into graphs and forms, open doors to scarce resources and give unquestionable evidence of quality within human services work.

In the next chapter, we expand on the incorporation of "beauty"—in the eyes of the bureaucratic beholder—into documents using graphs, charts, and other visuals. We have presented one example of such use in the current chapter: collected data that the youth fieldworker manager constrained and summarized in a series of graphs and charts presented on a display board. These elements add aesthetics to the magic of documents and serve to corral the uncertainty that can linger despite meticulous data collection and recording. As we show in the next chapter, the SIP offers a quintessential example of how this use of "beauty" gives rise to new documentation needs and a document superstructure, boosting the ongoing spiral of the *Eigendynamik*.

Notes

1 See, for example, https://english.alarabiya.net/en/News/world/2015/05/21/Sentence-extended-over-death-of-Palestinian-girl-in-Sweden (accessed 2021-02-05).
2 In Swedish: *Främjande samtal, Stödjande samtal,* or *Rådgivande samtal.*
3 In Swedish: Samordnad Individuell Plan (SIP).
4 See for example: https://www.ornskoldsvik.se/download/18.1c837f7a147e60b9ffb62241/1409060090643/Skriften+Samordnad+individuell+plan+-+decenniets+reform.pdf (Retrieved 2020/08/30).

6 Beauty and boost

In contrast to the common idea of paperwork as gray and dull, it can offer several pleasant and sought-after qualities, such as the beauty of displaying order and distinctness, of having something "in black and white." For example, templates, checklists, and flowcharts give a sense of orderliness that may be hard for human services workers (or anyone really) to experience or realize in their daily work. We saw an example of this in the preceding chapter when the manager of the field youth workers' office encapsulated years of inexact, ephemeral fieldwork into a series of charts and graphs for display.

The appealing powers of these documents tend to involve both their content and the graphic design. An organization chart, or "organigram" as it also is called, may express beauty in its simplicity and provide its designer with a creative challenge to depict order in a pleasant and aesthetic way. Presenting a slideshow is not only an occasion to pass on information or convey a message but also an opportunity to display creative skills. In this chapter, we continue the last chapter's discussion of the absorbing powers and pleasures of documents, but take it now from an aesthetic angle, examining how certain documents are boosted in the field of human services work.

Administrative tasks are seldom associated with aesthetic dimensions, but anthropologists have explored this link. Riles (1998) noted and examined the aesthetic appreciation of legal documents produced during UN conferences. Another example is Eggen (2012), who highlighted opportunities to present an image of a modern state and a professional bureaucracy through Malawi administrative procedures, no matter how ineffective. Yet another example is the Nigérian gendarmes (i.e., military police working in rural areas), whom Göpfert (2013) studied. The gendarmes invested both pride and professionalism in writing the "procès-verbal"—a legal crime report, subsequently sent to the prosecutor. First of all, the writing distinguished the gendarmes from the regular police, a difference the former often stressed. Second, they were concerned about producing beautiful documents because these would generate respect from both colleagues and their superiors. Göpfert (2013) claims that the striving for aesthetic

DOI: 10.4324/9781003108436-6

satisfaction is present among bureaucrats in many other fields globally and suggests that researchers explore this creativity. In our Swedish material from the human services sector, we have encountered similar expressions of what may count as bureaucratic beauty. Especially when complex and fuzzy work tasks are boiled down in a checklist or a schedule, professionals seem to appreciate the orderliness these documents provide.

Let us discuss the aesthetic aspects more specifically with the help of a particular type of document: the flowchart. A flowchart provides the opportunity to capture and materialize the process of a case in human services organizations, at least in standardized terms. These charts can be more or less elaborated, more or less colorful. Being skilled at producing flowcharts—or diagrams and graphs for that matter—may be a respected skill, highly valued by colleagues. It can be noted in comments in passing: "Wow! You're a pro!" when someone presents such efforts at a meeting. Or as a unit manager said encouragingly to an inferior: "Oh, you always do such nice documents with boxes and graphs!" Skills in drawing flowcharts and the like seem to be enviable, both for the (possibly) professional visual output and the ability to create order and clarity on paper.

Digital ease and aesthetics

Numerous software companies offer tools for creating administrative artwork that "looks professional." One of them offers: "Draw beautiful flowcharts easily and quickly with an online flowchart software." Another company urges users to "Make professional flowcharts in minutes," adding "It's super easy!" There are several colorful and ornated templates to choose from, some strict and businesslike and others more informal and imaginative—a service for professionals to use to create impressive and professional-looking flowcharts.

We have come across numerous examples of artistic flowcharts in the field. Below is a particularly colorful and detailed one, describing the process of incident reports filed at nursing homes. The colors indicate who is responsible for bringing the matter forward in the process and at what organizational level various kinds of reports should be handled. At times, as in this case, flowcharts seem to be overworked and particularly ornate, failing to produce the desired order and clarity. The flowchart below rather conveys the creator's joy in using colors, forms, and arrows to sort out the procedure. The shadows applied to the boxes have no particular function except to make the flowchart more appealing and artistic, or maybe they are added simply because the software made it possible (Image 6.1).

Visualizing quantitative and categorical information in graphs and charts can be viewed as a craft in itself, and the highly skilled chart constructors as Espeland and Stevens (2008:425) write about would likely dismiss this flowchart as "chartjunk" with "excessive use of color and pattern." The authors describe the strict technical and normative lessons taught by artful specialists in the graphical field who seek clarity and precision in their pictures. Such

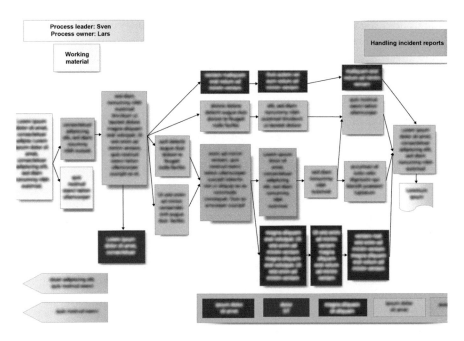

Image 6.1 Part of an elaborate and colorful flowchart describing the process of filing an incident report at a nursing home. The different colors indicate what organizational level should take action. The layout suggests care and a certain pleasure in constructing the flowchart. The text is translated/altered and partly blurred for anonymity reasons.

restrained, refined, and cultivated artistry has not yet reached the civil servants and professionals we have encountered, who happily if somewhat inexpertly use the flowchart to sort out all kinds of processes and procedures to create a visible order on paper.

As neat and organized as the described practices (or "processes") may seem in a flowchart, much effort is often invested in constructing them. Just as standardized instruments or classifications have a history of power struggles, disagreements, and compromises (Bowker and Leigh Star 1999), flowcharts are often preceded by negotiations. Below we analyze how a flowchart was created at a social services unit, showing a number of tensions and discussions underlying its production.

The absorbing power of a flowchart

Certain documents can be at the center of attention for long hours, involving many professionals, stimulating creative joy for producing neat and elegant (or not-so-neat and elegant) tables, schedules, and graphs during sometimes heated and emotional discussions. We find one such example from a social services unit where the drawing of a flowchart covering child welfare investigations turned into a series of weekly meetings with a handful participants. The unit's child welfare officers were obliged to participate in these meetings, and quite reluctantly did so initially, but eventually they became more and more involved. The flowchart project was initiated because of a large backlog of cases along with criticism from the Health and Social Care Inspectorate (IVO), which remarked that the unit's staff did not always follow the same procedures when informing clients about the investigation process. Furthermore, regulations regarding a "systematic quality work" from the Swedish National Board of Health and Welfare stipulate that the social services must identify, describe, and determine processes and routines to safeguard quality.[1]

The task, under the supervision of the quality coordinator Aina, was to picture the process from 1) when a complaint is filed to 2) when the child welfare officer reaches a decision, 3) possibly starts up an intervention or treatment of some kind, and finally 4) closes the case. A flowchart of this process was anticipated to improve efficiency, standardize work tasks, and make these tasks visual to service users through posting the flowchart on the community webpage.

The management decided that the whole child welfare team of about seven child welfare officers should come together with Aina to discuss the order of their work tasks. The project was sorted under headings such as "quality work," "development work," or "quality development." Ten times during the spring, about five child welfare officers (not always the same ones) had a 1.5-hour meeting. Fieldnotes from these ten meetings, totaling 15 hours, amounted to more than a hundred typed pages. The staff discussed the flowchart for the great majority of that time.

In the first four meetings, the team members discussed the child investigation process and simultaneously drew a flowchart together to visualize how families are investigated within the social services. In front of them at the table, there was a big sheet of paper, pens and markers, and sticky notes. With the help of example cases, child welfare officers discussed and negotiated how the common messiness of an investigation could be clarified and fit into boxes. The meetings were characterized by a fine-tuned struggle between Aina, the quality coordinator, who nudged the team members in a standardized direction, and the team members, who resisted this way of working, instead stressing the uniqueness of every case and the importance of flexible solutions for the case at hand.

During the first meetings regarding the flowchart, when the team members pointed out problematic or unforeseeable events, these were placed in a drawn "storm cloud" [*orosmoln*] on the paper, outside of the ordered process. The storm clouds were meant to symbolize concerns. Despite minor disagreements and some muttering about the time it took from other tasks, there was often a shared sense of accomplishment and satisfaction: "This is gonna be soooo good!" said one child welfare officer when they finished for the day.

Aina learned how to use a specific software program for constructing a flowchart that simplified the illustrations with boxes for the different parts of the process, and "storm clouds," where concerns or delays in the process were written down. At the fifth meeting, she demonstrated her new software skills and her efforts to summarize previous discussions into a digital flowchart. Before this meeting, she told the researcher that the program had facilitated her illustration tremendously and that it was "super smooth: you just click 'add' and then a new box shows up!" Aina placed a printed paper of the newly made flowchart on the table, said she had a few more questions, and asked the group to first take a moment to look at it.

The four child welfare officers present at the meeting made immediate cheerful comments when they viewed the flowchart: "Wow! How nice it looks!" (see Image 6.2). Aina explained that she has also considered the complaints put forward by the inspectorate (IVO) and that she has "synchronized the team's stories with the comments from the inspectorate." The subsequent five meetings were devoted to the presentation and revision of Aina's flowchart. It turns out that many of the detailed steps had to be erased because all unforeseeable things that may happen in individual cases could not

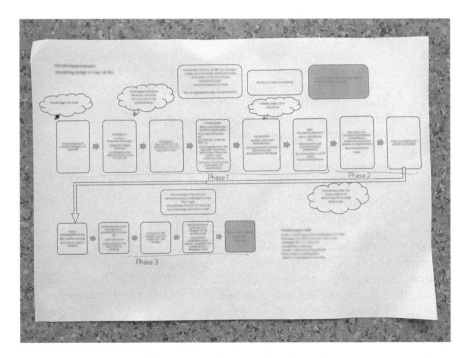

Image 6.2 Image boxes and "storm clouds" in Aina's flowchart when sketched using a digital program, based on the meetings with the child welfare officers. Concerns and uncertainties are placed in the storm clouds to keep the boxes' content as standardized as possible. The text is blurred for anonymity reasons.

be accounted for in the space the flowchart afforded. The team members concluded that the standard routines needed to be less specific. In line with this cutting-out practice, Aina's main concern had now become to remove the "storm clouds." In the version aimed for the control and management system, the flowchart could not be burdened with all the concerns and problems the team had identified. She says: "It should look more structured there, right?"

Even though the participants could agree on the beauty of an orderly and systematic description of the work process that grew out of their common efforts, Aina and the unit manager, Jenny, had to manage critique from team members about the very task of participating in meetings dominated by flowchart issues. Both Aina and Jenny were well aware of their understaffed situation and that the team members had a heavy workload. From time to time, Viveka, a child welfare officer, disclosed some discontent for investing so much time in the flowchart. At the final and tenth meeting, she is very explicit about it, and receives an equally explicit response from her superior, Jenny:

Viveka: I honestly think these team meetings are stressful. Honestly. Last week we spent two hours doing this. I would've had time to write a [child] investigation in those two hours. I have a much greater need to talk about cases. I'm just stressed by this. Mentally I am not really involved in this because I sit here and think about more acute cases.

Jenny: I fully understand that, but we can't avoid prioritizing this. In addition, we received criticism from IVO [the Health and Social Care Inspectorate], and we must do something about it. We have failed to prioritize this for years, and now we just have to deal with it, we cannot continue to blame other things. I will cling firmly to this development work.

This was the most evident critique and dismissive response visible in the field notes. More common from Aina and Jenny were "motivational pep talks." For instance, several reasons for why the child welfare officers should contribute to the flowchart construction were talked about: for their own sake (clarifying tasks and problems), for the sake of the inspectorate's critique, for the clients' sake, and for the sake of the newly hired employees. Another way of curbing criticism was to acknowledge the team's heavy burden while at the same time stressing that the members' input was indispensable. For example, Aina said: "I know you have so much to do with your cases and all, but without you this couldn't be done." Continuous pep talk could also be evaluative in positive terms with encouraging invitations for others to join in, as with Jenny here, the unit manager:

I'm happy with the discussions we have on the team meetings. It's good that we have time to discuss such things too, that we never do otherwise. I hope you have enjoyed it too.

Apart from this kind of motivational pep talk, there was another recurring conversational topic related to critique of the very idea of producing a flowchart: the repeatedly posed question, "What are we describing—wishful thinking or reality?" The question itself could partly be rhetorical, conveying disapproval. But at times it was posed as a sincere uncertainty: What were they talking about really? At the ninth meeting, the question is raised again by Misan, a child welfare officer:

Misan: Isn't the big question what we describe in the process charts? Is it how a dream situation looks like or what it actually looks like today? There is a huge difference, so I guess it's important that we know what it is to be described.
Malva: We started from the dream, what *should* be reasonable.
Aina: Yes, one has to think from a wishful point and describe the concerns in the clouds.

The result of the flowchart work was a digital picture of a far more neat and clean process than the handwritten paper that was developed during the first four gatherings. Messiness—complex and frequent exceptions associated with child investigations—were placed in the "storm clouds," which eventually were deleted from the final version.

How was the flowchart eventually used? As an example, it was presented at the "politicians day" when the social services met with politicians in the community. Aina is there to describe her quality work (i.e., producing the flowchart), and she presents the service-user as the flowchart's foremost beneficiary:

> – Say, for example, a report of a family to the Social Services: What happens and in what order? These are the processes we will describe. A school welfare officer may perhaps report a family, then she can click here [at the municipality web page] to see how the process goes and show it to the client. This creates security out there: you know what's going to happen. It's anxiolytic with detailed flows!
> Several of the politicians nod approvingly. One of them says:
> – It's also good that everyone is going in the same direction and doing the same thing.

The politician's comment, "Everyone is going in the same direction," suggests that the flowchart in itself guarantees that we now "do the same thing," which recalls the last chapter's theme of documents with a "touch of magic." The meeting participants seem to value the order visualized aesthetically in the flowchart. Put differently, the bureaucratic quest for order entails a particular appreciation of neat and clean charts.

Quite a few years after the flowchart meetings, the flowchart has still not been published on the municipality website. Instead, to our knowledge, it has been used in communication with politicians and in annual quality reports submitted to the controlling agency, IVO. The ambition to create a flowchart that provided clarity for the service-user seems to have been forgotten in the process.

What came out of these meetings? The results seem to rather nicely tie in to our theoretical starting point of an administrative *Eigendynamik*: more documents and meetings lie ahead. Apart from the flowchart itself, Aina promised to write templates for various situations to facilitate the child welfare officers' work. In addition, an area for improvement was identified: a group of workers will be assigned the task of going through and updating all pre-existing templates and decision formulations. "We thought about doing some formulations according to the laws that all can use," says Jenny, and the team members considered this helpful and needed. Aina has also realized that there are many more processes that need to be described in flowcharts (at least four): "There is a ripple effect," she concluded, another way to describe the self-perpetuating spiral.

Boosting up the SIP process

"A ripple effect," says the quality coordinator Aina, when she describes the need for more and more flowcharts to cover the organization's many "processes." Let's return to the care plan called SIP, that we discussed in the previous chapter, and examine a similar multiplying effect attached to documents. We start out by describing how this care plan was "boosted up" into a complex and important process, a necessary working tool for the benefit of the client or patient. The purpose with a SIP—a Coordinated Individual Plan—is to gather professionals from various agencies and have them agree on "who does what and when" for a particular patient or client present at the meeting. In other words, it is a contract on collaboration. If we recall the plain SIP form in Chapter 5 (Image 5.5), it is a fairly straightforward template, but it can still raise a number of questions.

This was the case at a manager meeting among the municipality's social services, preschools, and elementary school principals, where 11 participants discussed a variety of issues regarding the SIP. Some questions were utterly fundamental: What is a SIP really? What is the purpose? A school principal sounds very confident when stating that "The SIP is just a collection of documentation. It should be for support and help for the family. Not all families may need it because they keep track of things anyway." Others are more hesitant and expand on the name as such—"*A Coordinated Individual Plan*"—and want to explore how they all should "think about SIP" and what to call it. One social service manager suggests: "If saying 'my plan' or 'our plan in the family,' it gives a completely different feeling!" She indicates that "my plan" has a better ring to it than "SIP." Someone recommends a web link with a short film on "how to think about SIP." They also discuss procedural matters such as what agency should initiate a request for a SIP.

Not all questions were answered during this meeting. How could a fairly straightforward work procedure—planned collaboration, documented in a form—cause so much confusion and concern? Guided by the SIP buzz within the health care and social services, we decided to shadow the document itself (Jacobsson 2016), and we found evidence of a SIP document that is upscaled, packaged, and launched in elaborated ways, eventually described as the SIP *process.*

According to the instruction material, several steps precede the SIP meeting, as well as follow it—steps that are visualized in flowcharts to emphasize the processual quality of the invention. The many flowcharts to illustrate the SIP process are rather complex, and one flowchart is not like the other because municipalities and regions often make their own. Below is an example from the main implementing agent, the Swedish Association of Local Authorities and Regions (SALAR) and the project-based "Mission Psychiatric Health" (Image 6.3).

The brown boxes in the flowchart signal when documentation is deemed necessary, but let us focus on the blue boxes. The construction of the SIP in terms of a process is interesting for its emphasis on meetings rather than the realization of the planned and taken actions that the participants have agreed upon. Listing the central (blue) steps makes clear that the process is meticulously broken down, lingering on meeting-related topics:

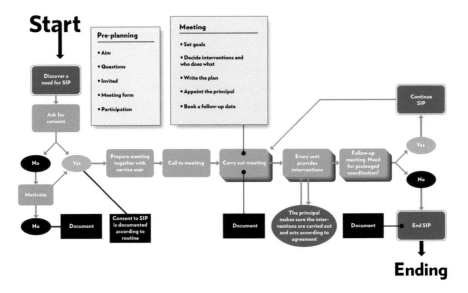

Image 6.3 A colorful illustration of the "SIP process" that has been revised and updated several times with different layouts, colors, and added boxes [our own translation].
Source: Mission Psychiatric Health at Swedish Association of Local Authorities and Regions (SALAR).

- Discovering a need for SIP
- Ask for consent (if no—motivate!)
- Prepare a meeting together with the service-user
- Call for a meeting
- Carry through the meeting
- All agencies provide interventions
- Follow-up meeting. Need for further cooperation?

If the answer is yes to the last question, it starts all over again. Meeting chains such as pre-meeting, meeting, and post-meeting are recognized from more organizations than only in the human services field (Hall, Leppänen, Åkerström 2019). In teaching materials for how to use a SIP, we also find advice, tips, and tools for how to carry through a SIP meeting. One of the early versions (third) includes an "Example of speech manuscript to support the meeting chairman" that is detailed to the letter with phrases and instructions. Below is an excerpt of the manuscript after half a page of welcoming and statements of the meeting's purpose. Spoken phrases are in italics, and instructions are in parentheses:

Excerpt from speech manuscript to support the chairman in a SIP meeting.[2]
"We have made an agenda for the meeting that looks like this."
(Write on the board or a paper so that all can see clearly)
"Now, we start with everyone introducing themselves as I don't think everyone has met before."
(Parents/relatives/child present themselves)
"Now the rest can introduce yourselves by name, what division you work for, and what contact you have with the child and the family."
(Representatives from each division present themselves and what contact they have with the family)/---/

In a later version of this teaching material (version 6),[3] the speech manuscript is replaced by meeting props that are promised to help in structuring the meeting. "The meeting circle can help create predictable and safe meetings," it says in the material, and "All participants get the same expectations of the meeting through the circle" (p. 68). Image 6.4 shows an example of a meeting circle aimed for the elderly.

Meeting circles are provided on the web under the heading "Print your own meeting circles" for professionals to download and cut out with a pair of scissors.[4] There is a separate meeting circle, marked by different colors, for all potential participant categories of the SIP meeting: Chairman, Youth, Parents, Adults, Elderly, Relatives, Staff, and finally the category Others. Each pie chart

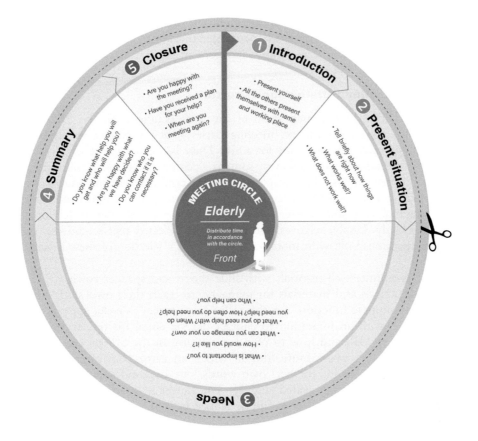

Image 6.4 The front page of an instructive "meeting circle," which works as a meeting prop for the elderly to use during a SIP meeting. The circle is meant to help structure the meeting and to assure that most of the time is spent on the service-user's needs. Circles of different colors are provided on the web for all categories of participants: "Print your own meeting circles!" [our translation] Source: Mission Psychiatric Health at Swedish Association of Local Authorities and Regions (SALAR).

contains instructions or questions for the participant to consider or ask during the various parts of the meeting: 1) Introduction, 2) Present situation, 3) Needs, 4) Summary, and 5) Closure. The design and size of the pie charts stipulates that half of the meeting should be spent on the service-user's concerns and needs. Users are instructed to make the meeting circles "synchronized" so that the participants can use them simultaneously.

The once plain SIP document ("who does what and when") has developed into a "process" that has to be explicated, learned, and mastered by professionals in human services organizations. The built-in meeting chain in dealing with the care plan SIP and the thorough instructions for how the

SIP meeting should be carried out signal a process of utmost importance. Taken together, they represent the building of a superstructure that has given a considerable boost to the new collaboration template launched and implemented by central and local management.

Building an administrative superstructure

We have already mentioned some of the side-documents to the SIP form (flowchart, speech manuscript, meeting circles) that are part of an administrative supportive superstructure for a SIP. There is much more to discover. In fact, the remarkable production of support documents and other educational means seems endless. The employer organization SALAR provides a tremendous amount of material on their websites. Apart from handbooks, teaching materials, and information targeting every possible category (children, youth, elderly, family, relatives, professional, and elected representatives), the superstructure is built with more material. Below, a selection of these is listed:

- Sixty-minute web tutorials with slide shows and speaker voices.
- Instructions and materials for managers to teach their own staff.
- The "support function" for the SIP: "Ask Viveka!" Viveka appears in a picture with an invitation to contact her via email for tips and advice regarding SIPs and how to plan for a course in the SIP process.
- Vignettes—a two-minute film in which an actor performs a service-user's story "in his [or her] own words." In a second subsequent film, the situation is aggravated slightly. The viewer is asked to reflect upon whether the service-user would be helped by a SIP, and if the worsened situation could have been avoided if a SIP had been established in the first place. Stories of five service-users of varying ages and genders are dramatized.
- Animated instruction video: "SIP in three minutes!"
- Videos in which service-users (or family members) tell about their life situation and how things now work fine since they got a SIP. Voices from managers, nurses, case workers, or other staff confirm that SIP is vital for the service-user's well-being and sense of security.
- One-page interviews in stylish layouts with service-users or their relatives, with headlines such as "SIP was a relief to me" and "I would've needed a SIP!"
- Case descriptions with related questions about whether a SIP should be established and who is responsible.

In addition, a website named "The SIP check" [sipkollen.se] provides a digital evaluation survey for clients to fill out under the headline, "We want to know how you experienced having a SIP." The respondent first ticks the boxes for age, gender, region, and municipality, and eventually encounters the following statements to agree or disagree with using a Likert scale:

I think the staff listened to me.

I am involved and get to decide on what support I or my family should receive.

I think we talked about things that are important to me.

I think it is clear who does what.

I think I got my questions answered.

Regardless of age and mental capabilities, the service user is asked to tick the happy or sad faces to express degree of agreement with the statement (see Image 6.5).

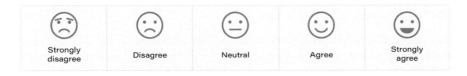

Image 6.5 A digital "customer survey" for service-users to fill in after their first SIP, gathered for the production of statistics and national comparisons. [our translation] Source: www.sipkollen.se.

On the website, it is also possible to view graphs depicting how happy service users are with SIPs on average nationally (very happy), and a top-ten list for the municipalities (social services) and regions (health care) that use SIP most frequently per every hundred thousand inhabitants. We learn that Uppsala municipality is outstanding in this respect. The manual for how to generate statistics tailored to dates and regions reveals how to do it step by step.

SALAR also makes sure that manuals, teaching materials, and handbooks are updated. For example, the previously mentioned *Use SIP—a tool for collaboration. Children and Youth 0–18 years* can now be found in its sixth version. Compared with the third version of around 50 pages, the sixth version comes in a more appealing layout and contains twice as many pages: almost 100 pages divided into 15 chapters and 4 appendices. In this latest version, some years have passed since the introduction of the SIP—enough time for critical opinions of the SIP to be formulated. Such voices are dealt with in an explicit manner under the heading, "Myths about SIP." Three statements are listed:

"SIP is difficult."

"SIP takes time."

"SIP should only be used in complex cases."

Each statement—framed as a "myth"—is refuted effectively. The answer to those who think it is difficult to go through with the SIP process is short and sharp: "Meeting and agreeing on who should do what and when does not have to be difficult." It is hard not to consider this answer contradictory to the growing superstructure around SIP that indeed indicates that SIP is at least challenging and demanding, if not rocket science. The section ends with questions for the learners to discuss: "What myths about SIP have you encountered?" and "How do you work with these myths?" The strategy of "soft regulation" comes to mind: the subtle transformation of practices with the help of a common language use and shared knowledge making, as Kerstin Jacobsson (2004) found when she studied the EU employment policy. However, there is nothing subtle with the SIP persuasion campaign we have studied. Efforts to convince users of this document's superiority come across as rather forceful and blunt.

The multiplying effect of a care plan

The myriad activities associated with the introduction of the SIP and the multiplying effect are even more visible in the fact that each municipality and city council constructs their own handbooks, checklists, teaching materials, and manuals. The SIP form and the material adherent to it are tailored to the specific service areas and client categories. Although the basic outline is very similar, a SIP may vary with age ("Children and youth" vs. "Adults") and client category (e.g., psychiatric patients, the elderly). Furthermore, the teaching material is adjusted according to the target group: "ordinary staff" or managers and directors.

Paradoxically, efforts to standardize a working tool give rise to numerous local routines to make the standard fit with local circumstances, creating what we called in the first chapter "confusion yet to be ordered." Thus, more ordering is required, perpetuating the process. The SIP care plan is further often digitalized with an advanced communication system for the professional actors to use when "calling" on each other for requesting a plan and deciding when to hold the meeting. Also, the client's consent is to be registered in the digitalized "plan system." Accordingly, another document—for example, the 64-page "User manual for my plans"[5]—concerns all technical details for how to navigate in the computerized system. The many municipalities and regions have their own user manuals because they use different systems.

This process clearly fits the concept of administrative *Eigendynamik* (Simmel 1904/1957). Attempts to create order and clarity always hold some degree of vague instructions or uncertainties, which in turn generate the need for more clarity and order. Ambiguity needs to be addressed and sorted out with new checklists, flowcharts, or manuals. Correspondingly, the administrative superstructure for the SIP continues to grow. The range of support is difficult to encompass or use, even by the professionals. Some municipalities have now established positions such as SIP coordinator (also called SIP coach or SIP supporter), whose role is different from the professional who is responsible for the SIP plan. But one might wonder what it is that a SIP coordinator does. It turns out that there is a checklist for this, too.[6] Examples of a SIP coordinator's work tasks may be to develop documentation for the SIP or proposals for local guidelines and templates. And so the self-perpetuating administrative spiral continues.

Conclusion

More and more, administrative skills in terms of handling meetings and producing documents are included in the specific *esoteric knowledge*, as Hughes (1963) puts it, that is claimed by a profession. For example, managers within the Swedish social services may be discontent with newly graduated social workers' lack of detailed knowledge in the documentary system for the day. A three- to four-day course on how to document a child investigation can be given disproportionate emphasis considering years of social work education at the university.

The upgrading and embrace of administrative skills in human services professions are further visible in a conspicuous preoccupation with detailed guidelines for having meetings and filling out documents, and the appreciation of beauty in these practices.

The vast production and expansion of SIP-related documents discussed in this chapter suggests a technical (hyper)engagement with the documents (or their system) per se. It seems obvious that this kind of "meta-documentation"—the production of documents *about* a particular way of documenting clients' needs (in this case)—demands a great amount of labor and effort. The meta-documentation itself (from authorities, managers, controllers, etc.) signals that this "tool" is of utmost importance, thus demanding attention from professionals. Attempts to standardize working methods, such as "collaboration," generate a bulging workload with the risk of causing competition—or confusion—between "doing the document" and "doing the doing" (Ahmed 2007), such as talking to, treating, or helping clients and patients. The task of doing the documents may be rewarding enough because it signals good performance in a more visible and concrete way than the work of carrying out "interventions," which often involves vague or uncertain outcomes. But the result is an endless administrative spiral.

Another source of competition that can contribute to this spiral arises among the organizations that are expected to collaborate on such documentation. This competition in itself can be a meeting and documentation generator as tensions build about details, division of labor, and conflicts over time spent on "doing the document" vs. "doing the doing." As we examine in the next chapter, these tensions and the back-and-forth that such competition generates contribute to the continuation of the administrative *Eigendynamik*.

Notes

1 SOSFS 2011:9. Ledningssystem för systematiskt kvalitetsarbete. [Management system for systematic quality work]. The Swedish National Board for Health and Welfare. https://www.socialstyrelsen.se/globalassets/sharepoint-dokument/artikelkatalog/foreskrifter-och-allmanna-rad/2011-6-38.pdf [Retrieved 2020-09-29].

2 Använd SIP—ett verktyg vid samverkan. Barn och unga 0–18 år. (Version 3). [Use SIP—a tool for collaboration. Children and Youth 0–18 years. (Version 3). Issued by Psychiatric Health, children and youth, p. 43. https://www.ystad.se/globalassets/dokument/soc/anvandsip_digital3mars.pdf [Retrieved 2020-09-15].

3 Använd SIP—ett verktyg vid samverkan. Barn och unga 0–18 år. (Version 6.0). [Use SIP—a tool for collaboration. Children and Youth 0–18 years. (Version 6.0). Issued by SALAR. https://www.uppdragpsykiskhalsa.se/wp-content/uploads/2020/04/Använd-SIP-Ett-verktyg-för-samverkan-0-till-18-år-vers-6.0.pdf [Retrieved 2020-09-15].

4 https://www.uppdragpsykiskhalsa.se/sip/sip-mote/motescirkel/skriv-ut-egna-motescirklar/ [Retrieved 2020-08-20].

5 For example: http://vardgivare.skane.se/siteassets/6.-it/it-stod-och-tjanster/mina-planer-svplsip/anvandarmanual-mina-planer-ver-1.5.pdf [Retrieved 2019-01-20. No longer open but requires log in and identification from staff working at the region.]

6 https://www.uppdragpsykiskhalsa.se/wp-content/uploads/2018/10/Checklista-för-SIP-samordnare.pdf [Retrieved 2020-09-17].

7 Spirals of meetings and documents

It would seem easy to recognize that documents and meetings are interrelated. A written agenda is sent out before a meeting, and afterwards meeting minutes are written. The sequence *agenda–meeting–minutes* is taken for granted in today's organizations. It is institutionalized and somehow perpetuates itself. Minutes are routinely taken, even in contexts where a summarized record seems irrelevant, as when one of our interviewees muttered, leaving a team-meeting: "Who will *use* them? Nothing was even decided."

This integration of meetings and documents is thus in a very basic way routinely institutionalized in the administrative world of contemporary organizations, but few researchers have actually studied in what ways. In *Handbook of Meeting Studies* (ed. by Allen et al. 2015), Schwartzman (2015:743) calls for precisely such study: to "begin to consider and theorize the relationship that exists between meetings and documents."

In the previous chapters, we focused on either meetings or documents, but we have also seen how the production of documents involves meetings and vice versa, especially with our example of the SIP (a Coordinated Individual Plan) in the preceding chapter. In this chapter, we will explicitly discuss how meetings and documents generate each other in profound and multiple ways. We will particularly analyze one case—a youth care project—where documents were put in the foreground, discussed, and contested during meetings.

An interplay of order and disorder

When Schwartzman (2015) calls for investigations of the interplay between meetings and documents, she touches on a theme we highlighted in Chapter 1: accelerating administrative efforts can be seen as part of a self-propelling process between order and disorder. Schwartzman's allusion to order and disorder as an important research theme references contentious issues and efforts to solve them through meetings. Indeed, in her work, she relies on a study of a meeting-intense context: an alternative health organization where staff's discussions centered on how to best pursue health. She describes various conflicts and unclear situations that the staff tried to solve through new meetings.

DOI: 10.4324/9781003108436-7

Although Schwartzman noted this trait in relation to meetings, we can see the same pendulum swings when it comes to documents. As examples in the previous chapter show, documents and meetings may be arranged in the hope of bringing order and clarity but can themselves generate new issues or situations that appear disorderly. Disorder may be created by questioning a document or a meeting or introducing new ones so that organizational members no longer go about their work in relation to taken-for-granted administrative routines. Perceived disorder may in turn bring about new efforts "from below" consisting of new meetings or in creating new documents to resolve conflicts, clarify the unclear, or bring structure into a messy reality. In short, an administrative *Eigendynamik* is generated.

Meetings and documents between them also can create their own self-perpetuating spiral. Conflicts may arise in relation to meetings, and in such conflicts, documents might become important tools for easing tensions. In an article on the World Health Organization, Nicolas Lamp (2017) describes a critique that decisions were made in more informal small meetings between powerful groups. For the sake of increased transparency, there were demands to make documents related to these meetings available. These demands resulted in one of the participant's going around the conference room after a negotiation session and collecting notes left by the delegates. These notes were then archived electronically (Lamp 2017:73) and eventually published in the form of working papers or as "room documents." In other words, conflicts concerning informal meetings were solved through practices concerning documents.

On the other hand, problems may start with documents and be solved through meetings. One such example is given by the Swedish anthropologist Renita Thedvall (2019) in a study of an "activation policy" of the unemployed. Human services workers from different organizations handled four documents that were supposed to fit like cogs one after the other in an ostensibly efficient process, but the process lacked the expected flow. One interviewee in Thedvall's study explained that they had hoped for a smooth routine when they mapped it out in a simple logical way, but "this was one and a half years ago, she said, and since then we have been working to make it operational" (Thedvall 2019:223). During meetings, some of the problems with division of labor were identified and resolved. Meetings in this case thus functioned as "smoothing machines" among the professionals who represented different organizations, easing conflicts about how they would work with the documents.

To study the multilayered interplay between meetings and documents, here we investigate one case in more detail: a youth care project. In contrast to the examples described previously in which conflicts can be solved either through meetings or through documents, our case shows how a struggle can be kept alive with the help of both meetings and documents. A common sociological assumption from Simmel's (1964) analyses of conflicts is that the more intimate a relationship is, the more intense conflict will be. We suggest that the intimate relationship is not only in the web of relations in the human services world but also in their relations to administrative objects and events.[1]

A youth care project's meetings and documents

We will mainly use an illustration gathered from a youth care project to illustrate both how meetings and documents are tightly connected and how such administrative concerns can be generated from below (Åkerström 2019; Åkerström and Wästerfors, forthcoming). The case concerns one of the most expensive governmental projects in Swedish youth care, when the Swedish National Board of Institutional Care was tasked with designing a strengthened "care chain" in relation to young people with psychosocial problems, substance abuse, and criminal behavior. This governmental organization was to take on this project in cooperation with the social authorities in 15 Swedish municipalities. A project leader and a small administrative team were chosen, and they employed 24 coordinators. The project team also arranged a central reference group, as well as five local reference groups that were geographically close to the municipalities. The coordinators worked in five cities in offices rented for this purpose. The municipality got a fee reduction of 40% when placing young people in detention homes if they also assigned them to the project.

The coordinators, all social workers, were intended to act as facilitators or coordinators for the young people. They each were assigned between 20–25 youths, and their job was to ensure that when the youths were released from youth care institutions, post-care plans were enacted, such as suitable school placements or work training. Even if the coordinators' tasks were supposed to concentrate on aftercare, the project was set up so that they had already met the young person in the detention home and attended meetings there to be able to help with the client's future planning.

During this process, the coordinators were expected to keep in close contact with the youths and their families. The project changed, however, to become more and more administrative. The coordinators spent more time in various meetings with other professionals and less with the youths. It was significant that the youths were designated by a first name—Joseph, Camilla, Mustafa, and so on—in the beginning, but later were referred to as "cases" by the coordinators. The coordinators became more and more occupied with documents, to the extent that the youths saw the coordinators as peripheral actors: one of them, for instance, asked the fieldworker if the coordinators were "the ones sending documents"? Furthermore, the coordinators became involved in a *document struggle* often enacted during meetings with the co-operating partners—representatives for the social services and staff at the detention homes.

Here, we will follow this project in relation to its meetings and documents and focus especially on how one document, *The Agreement*, was invented and authored by the project members and how this document produced a lot of tension within the project and in relation to its colla-borating organizations. These tensions were aired during the many meetings that were held. The two tables below give an overview of the project's meetings and documents (Tables 7.1 and 7.2).

Table 7.1 Types of meetings.

Names of meetings	Meetings that refer to each other
Work group meeting	The last meeting
Extra meeting	Previous meetings
Pre-meeting	The next meeting
Group meeting	Future meetings
Information meeting	Meetings as references to various categories of people
Registration meeting	Meetings with social services
Local work group meeting	Meetings with parents etc.
Admission meeting	Old and new forms
Planning meeting	Video meetings are distinguished from "ordinary
Midpoint meeting	meetings"
Handover meeting	Words and phrases that indicate place, time, or rhythm
Follow-up meeting	Meeting rooms
Network meeting	Meeting frequency
Personnel meeting	Meeting times
Reference group meeting	Monday meeting
Recommendation meeting	Friday meeting
Coordinate coordinators meeting	
School meeting	
"Soc" (social services) meeting	
Team meeting	
Breakfast meeting	
Telephone meeting	
Assignment meeting	
Weekly meeting	
Video meeting	

From Åkerström (2019:56).

Table 7.2 Documents referred to in the youth project.

Name of document	Name of document (contd.)
The Agreement (the project's)	Evaluation of project questionnaire
Care Plan (social authorities)	Evaluation of treatment in detention homes
Treatment Plan (detention homes)	Social network maps
Implementation plan	Journals
Information about the project	School evaluations
Psychological evaluation	Reports about the projects
IQ tests	Steering document
Client records	Letters
Family evaluation	

The meetings collected various social categories and were accompanied by different documents. Many of the meetings were not required by "top-down" demands. The project leaders organized a central reference group as well as several local reference groups that met regularly. Such groups were not required, but initiated by the project leader presumably as they belong to the taken-for-granted ways of "doing projects" in human service organizations. And the coordinators suggested new meetings themselves: "Coordinating coordinators," and "Team meetings." The latter were weekly meetings of small groups, varying from four to five people, in their rented apartment (functioning as an office), which made the field researcher wonder why they did not simply talk when meeting each other on a more or less daily basis. The coordinators also complained about lack of time but insisted on attending scheduled meetings at the detention homes, which the project leader instead tried to minimize because the project's focus was meant to be on the aftercare. The documents circulated in the project derived from detention homes and the social authorities, but the project participants also produced their own steering documents, brochures, evaluations, and reports, apart from The Agreement.

Getting started: turning disorder into order

The project leaders were given generous financing but not very clear directives on how to arrange the project. So how would they go about this? In the first meetings where all of the coordinators were gathered to discuss how to organize their work, one of them came up with the idea of producing a document, *The Agreement* (in Swedish: *Överenskommelsen*), which would pinpoint in detail what the youth wanted and needed such as school courses, work practice, and leisure activities. We will return to this document in more detail below, and it will be the main focus of the remainder of this chapter.

Another "invention" was tied to meetings that concerned the youth, where the social services and staff from detention homes would participate. The coordinators were expected to "take over" those meetings by acting as chairs. By being chair, they could make suggestions, remind others such as social workers or detention home staff, and through "soft power" hold them accountable if they had not executed what they had promised.

The satisfaction, even relief and happiness, were palpable when the project leader commented on these ideas in a short interview at the end of the meeting. By deciding on two administrative tools: coordinators serving as chairs and constructing The Agreement, they had solved the issue of how to proceed, using both meetings and documents as their solution. Now, he said, they knew how to work. These decisions thus promised to create order in a situation where routines, plans, and strategies were not yet settled. Now they could produce a document, a brochure, that could be used to explain the project to outside audiences and to the government that had financed the project. And they had established a plan for meetings and who would serve as chairs.

All of the coordinators were experienced human services workers and could be expected to be especially competent because they had gotten their job in a tough competition. Their assignment was clear in that it consisted of helping the youth who had been involved in some criminality through making concrete plans together with their parents about, for example, schools, work, and leisure activities. One could expect the coordinators to be confident about how to perform without any particular governing details regarding how to accomplish their assignment. However, when the co-ordinators had worked for a short while and were installed in their office, they gathered for a so-called team meeting and criticized the projects' lack of organization and directives. For instance: a written detailed work description is missing!

> Inga says she has become very frustrated by the lack of structure in the project. "I will honestly say that in fact I actually thought of quitting," she says with a serious tone and leans forward in the chair. "There's been a lot of problems and hassle," she says, adding to the complaints of the others, Peter, Gahlib, and Cecilia, who have voiced their criticism earlier in the meeting. They have pointed to the lack of routines and how much they have had to work out on their own. They have not received a detailed job description from the project management.

The researchers in the project later reflected on their consternation because human services workers often complained about bureaucracy and rules, hindering them from doing professional work (Hall et al. 2006; Goldman and Foldy 2015). Why did they complain about the lack of a detailed work description? Why didn't they go about their business with confidence? Why weren't they grateful even for being able to use their own professional judgment and the tools, experience, knowledge, and network they had gathered in previous stages of their career? The answer, we would suggest, can be found in the ontological insecurity that this relative freedom provides. Documents with detailed job instructions seem to provide the reassurance of a predictable framework in which to both perform and evaluate one's tasks.

Adding to existing documents

Along with The Agreement and the job description, another document was discussed early on, one that outlined the project: "The role of the co-ordinator in the care chain project youth-MVG" (SiS 2006).[2] According to some project members, this document did not properly and clearly explicate the project's goals. In the beginning of the project, one of the coordinators, Susanne, tells the researcher who is accompanying her during a workday that the formulation "Achieving positive and lasting changes for the young people" in this document is too vague:

She shows me the document and explains that the goals for their work are vague. She wants to break down the general goals to "sub-aims" and concrete work tasks. "For example: What should the coordinator do during an emergency placement, investigation, or treatment?"

Susanne describes that she has started to formulate a new document that is more precise than the original. Furthermore, she complains about her team not getting enough time to meet other coordinators (who are placed in different regions). During such a meeting, the participants could discuss the new document and form a collective understanding of how exactly they should work for "achieving positive and lasting changes for the young people."

Eventually, plans were made for a meeting with all the coordinators, a meeting labeled "Coordinating coordinators." The team we followed especially closely looked forward to these meetings and their hopes were high: maybe that meeting as well as formulating a new document would create routines and shared understandings of what their work tasks should consist of? When all of the coordinators actually met, they rewrote the document that outlined the project. Their attempt to produce a unifying document was thus successful, holding promises of shared order. However, the formulations that the coordinators agreed upon were later contested after being presented at a local reference group meeting.

Participants in this meeting consist of managers from the social services, managers from youth detention homes, the project leader, and Inger, a representative for the coordinators. When the meeting reached the point of discussing the document, Inger explained that the coordinators had all agreed on some principles, and she read aloud from a document:

> "A plan shall be established for the care of the young, and the young person and the family must participate in the establishment of the plan." Astrid, a manager from the social services, disagrees immediately, stating that the coordinators cannot provide directives to them. She says: "Naturally, we strive for as much participation as possible, but there may be reasons why this may not be possible in some cases. So I object to the formulation 'must.'" Inger says that this was the formulation given in the government's directive for the project, but Astrid is still not convinced.

It does not help that Inger, the coordinator, refers to the government's directive. The conflict is not solved during the meeting. Moreover, as mentioned earlier, documents may create strong emotional involvement. In this case, outside the meeting frame, the situation developed into a conflict between the coordinator and the project leader as Inger claims that the project leader had not mustered a defense for the coordinators' suggestion. The next day, Inger left work on sick leave.

Anchoring processes

A tendency that increases administrative efforts in terms of meetings and documents is visible when something new is introduced into an old and stable organization. Projects are one such element, increasingly used in the public sector (Hodgson et al. 2019). They are new temporary organization, with new demands and new people, and must be inserted among old routines. In many organizations, such initiatives demand "an anchoring process," that is, to get everyone on board. We can see not only how such efforts are being done in the project by the coordinators arranging information meetings (see the discussion of The Agreement) but also how a discussion of anchoring takes place, a sort of meta-commentary among the project members.

We are now placed in a new local reference meeting taking place in a conference room at a detention home. The meeting starts, and the floor goes to Inez (a coordinator), who points out that there are still ambiguities about how the coordinators work with the detention homes and the social services. She complains about how staff at one detention home had refused to open the document "Aftercare Act," which was necessary for her to be able to document the aftercare of a discharged youth in the computer system. The project manager says that he has written to all detention homes about this, so that no such problems should arise in the future. But the information and anchoring process has to go on! A social services manager says that there is still anchoring work going on—she has received indications that not all of her social workers are on board. The same goes for the detention homes, where it is said that the issue will be raised again at a regional council as a way of anchoring everyone.

> The project manager says that it's great that these things come up, "that's exactly what these meetings are for." Hedda from the social services believes that it's perfectly normal with some run-in problems in a new project, that it's searching for its way right now and has to be allowed to take some time. Danny [a coordinator] points out that now you have to start from what exists and work with regular information and anchoring. Katja, head of the detention home in the southern region, agrees and says that one should not have too high expectations at the beginning of the project, "there's always a need for anchoring, we might have to keep it up until the end of the project."

This meeting took place after the coordinators had worked for at least four months, and the project as a whole was ten months old (the projected lasted for three years). Still, the meeting members refer to the project as "new" and moreover expect that an anchoring process is necessary before really getting it off the ground. Such anchoring processes imply more meetings and the delivery of documents to different units in various organizations. In the everyday work life of the detention homes and in the social workers' work lives, projects are coming and going, apart from the myriad tasks. Moreover, newcomers in the different organizations are ignorant of the project, which also suggests that the anchoring process should be kept alive. In a hierarchal organization in another time, such anchoring work would perhaps not be required. As van Vree (2011) has observed, the "meetingization" in contemporary western societies is propelled by an increased mutual dependency among different organizations as well an increasing democratization, where different parties are supposed to be coordinated, involved, and have their say.

Solving tensions with meetings?

At times, tensions concerning documents can be resolved through meetings, as mentioned earlier (Thedvall 2019). In the youth project, we could observe that the mere *suggestion* of meetings could be used to smooth out differences, if such suggestions are interpreted as constructive proposals.

Going back to the local reference group meeting, where the coordinators' reformulation of the project's goal was discussed: "A plan shall be established for the care of the young, and the young person and the family must participate in the establishment of the plan." Earlier, the formulation of "must" was questioned. After a while, the discussion returns to the wording in the proposed document: now, it is "participate" that is questioned. The social services manager, Astrid, turns to Inez, the representative for the coordinators, and asks: "What do you mean, for example, with participate? We have semantic problems here between the social authorities and SiS [the authority who organizes the detention homes], we mean different things."

At this point, Karin, who is the head manager at the youth detention home where the meeting takes place, suggests that perhaps they should try to arrange a research seminar. Another participant, Johan, proposes that representatives from detention homes and the social services have different cultures and that they therefore should meet and get to know each other in more relaxed forms. The others are positive. The discussion is closed with the project leader's mentioning video conferencing as a way to increase the family's participation when the young person is placed far away from home. At this point, the struggle about the wording in the document ends with the suggestion of not one but three different types of meetings: research seminar, a "get-together" meeting, and video conferences. Meeting suggestions thus seem to be an item that can dilute conflicts and align members temporarily as long as they are interacting inside the meeting frame.

Embracing "The Agreement": making it ours

As was mentioned earlier, The Agreement would pinpoint in detail the young person's future plans and needs. The document should also state who should do what: the youths themselves, treatment assistants, parents, the social services, school representatives, or coordinators. In this way, each of the participating parties could be held accountable if they had failed to do what was agreed upon when they met again in upcoming meetings.

After the decision to construct The Agreement, the idea was followed up in coordinators' subsequent meetings where they built up arguments in support of this document. One of the ways of "beefing it up" was by contrasting The Agreement with the other documents, such as the treatment plan used by detention homes. From an early "team meeting" with four of the coordinators:

Peter: Detention homes state that everyone has an individual treatment plan, but in reality they don't. /---/ it seems that everyone has the same treatment plan, where I've worked. Besides, this [The Agreement] certifies that, when we set up the goals or sub-goals, these are the ways things have to be done. /---/

Cecilia: And it's really important that everyone agrees. That everyone has decided this together. Then, everyone knows what applies and that it becomes a common goal with the youth in focus. That's important, I think.

Anne: As for responsibility: each one comes aboard, and it will be like we're all partners. *That's* the thing that's decided and what everyone is responsible for in aftercare. And then no one can say that this is not my responsibility. You've got to work together for the best of the young ones!

Hedda: I just think that the detention homes' treatment plans are really based on the evaluation units there. /---/

Cecilia: It is an *evaluation plan* and there we have the difference [compared to The Agreement].

Hedda: Then they call that a treatment plan, but I don't know … (shaking her head)

By questioning the detention homes' treatment plan, they arrive somewhat triumphantly at the conclusion that it is "really" (only) "an evaluation." Supposedly, the label "evaluation" implies that this deals with the youth's past problems and a diagnosis of these, whereas The Agreement was based on planning the future. Moreover, it is claimed that the detention homes' document is not customized: "In reality it is the same for all." In this way, the coordinators gather and unite around their own document. The discussion also made clear that they envisioned the power of the document as creating orderliness to their own work: goals would be created for the youths, and by uniting on the formulations, "everyone" would come aboard, and no one would be able to escape their responsibility.

Document struggles

The Agreement promised order but created disorder because it was contested by other professionals. It generated a document competition and gave rise to competence criticism, struggles about work divisions, and internal struggles about how to manage the document: when it was supposed to be written and by whom.

The coordinators' commitment to The Agreement continued to be strong throughout the project, but other professional representatives such as staff at detention homes and at the social services questioned the document. Such criticism could take up quite a bit of meeting time. The fight over the documents can be described as a *document competition.* The social services had their care plan, and the detention homes had their treatment plan.

Representatives from these organizations raised concerns that The Agreement could collide with, duplicate, or interfere with existing documents that they themselves used. These other professionals described The Agreement as unnecessary and increasing the workload, viewing it as a symptom of bureaucratization of their work. These discussions were held in many of the meetings we attended.

Consider, for instance, an information meeting at the beginning of the project. This meeting was initiated by a team of coordinators and was intended to present the project for managers from the social services in their region. Early on in the meeting, one of the social services managers questions The Agreement by stating that they already had their own document: the care plan. "I foresee a high risk of confusion!" Despite the coordinators' explanations, the manager insists: "I still think it's confusing." Other managers agree, and the atmosphere becomes tense. The coordinators try to explain the advantages of their document and the differences between the two documents, but the social services managers are not convinced. This information meeting generates a new meeting: back at their office, the coordinators hold a team meeting where they discuss the morning meeting with the social services and agree that they have to polish their arguments before participating in or arranging new information meetings.

Cooperation among different organizations demands *diplomacy* before, during, and after meetings (Hall, Leppänen, and Åkerström 2019). The project leader illustrates this when the document was discussed during reference group meetings. In one such case, a social services manager points out that their care plan is used when the county court is involved in deciding that someone has to stay for a period in a detention home. She asks what the difference is in relation to The Agreement, and furthermore, who "owns" the document?

> The project leader pointed out that the task of the coordinators is not to replace already functioning routines with others, but rather to provide help, advice, and support. He also talked about the "power of the

question": Will the young person speak, will his or her interests be safeguarded? Could anything be better? Has this been done? According to the project leader, The Agreement should not be seen as something that replaces the care plan but as a complement to it. He also pointed out that the responsibility for the young person remains with the social service; no formal power has been transferred to the coordinators. If the care plan is complete and good, no other agreement is really needed, which was the project leader's conclusion.

The diplomatic efforts were not quite successful; some frustration and comments were expressed in the style of "but I *still* don't understand what you mean" and "but then I just have to add" and so on.

It was not only the social services that engaged in the competition struggle, defending their care plan. Representatives from the detention homes (who had the treatment plan) were also annoyed by the project's Agreement. When the project coordinators talk about the project, and mention The Agreement at a meeting with a detention home manager, he expresses his doubts: "When there already exists this type of document, the one we have (the treatment plan), I don't think you need to create another document on top of the other." The comment is expressed with some emphasis.

The coordinators, in turn, related conflicts with the social services or the detention homes during their own meetings and in talking to the field observers. One coordinator complained for instance that: "They don't want to understand, but think that the care plan (from the social services) is enough ---- But the care plan is not concrete as our Agreement, it's very general and intended to be used for the court (when youths are taken into care)."

The coordinators did not confine their complaints to other professionals' resistance towards their document. Their own criticisms towards representatives from the organizations they collaborated with also could become quite harsh. Sometimes, the criticism was expressed in ironic words in which a competency competition becomes clear, and this could be focused on others' lack of knowledge. Consider, for instance, the statement from one of the coordinators towards the end of the project when the team gathered to evaluate the project. Some staff from the social services are said to be incompetent, which, one claims, is clearly visible in their inability to tell one document from another:

> But I mean, when it [criticism] comes from a social welfare office where they don't know the difference between care plans and treatment plans. Then you get scared!... At the same time, they think that they're incredibly competent... (ironic tone of voice)

Document struggles were not exclusively turned against the other professionals. The Agreement gave rise to disputes among the coordinators as well.

This was the case when discussing *when* it was to be introduced and *who* would write it. At a breakfast meeting, the coordinators discussed at what time in the treatment process The Agreement should be written.

> It's agreed that the document will be filled in when the young people are enrolled in the detention home. The three coordinators argue against the stance taken by an absent coordinator [who wants to do the document when the youth is enrolled in the project]. One of them says irritably: "I don't really understand how she thinks. We have to wait until soc [the social services] finds a suitable detention home and have made their decisions."

Each of the team of coordinators in different regions developed slightly different work routines and policies. One issue concerned not only when but also *who* was to write the document. Discussions centered on the division of labor between social services staff and the coordinators in relation to writing The Agreement. Initially, the coordinators were responsible for this. But eventually some coordinators wanted the social workers employed by the social services to fill in The Agreement. According to one of the co-ordinators, this practice had led to a struggle among the different regions.

Anna:　　　　There has been a war between us [in the different regions].
Interviewer:　Having their own variants?
Anna:　　　　Yeah… Then we ask the project manager: "you choose," between different variants. He does. But then they [the North region] don't give a damn.

"There has been a war between us" is strong wording. The "war" was played out at meetings among colleagues, as when all coordinators were gathered in a "coordinating the coordinators meeting" where the project leader also got a side-swipe of the whip as he was charged with not being firm enough with the wrongdoers.

The issue of who was responsible for filling in the document seems to be given a symbolic boundary in relation to professional duties (Lamont and Molnár 2002; Allen 2000). In a team meeting, the coordinators construct the practice of filling in The Agreement as a task belonging to the exercising of public authority that only social workers are allowed to do.

Patricia:　　And yet we are asked (by the social services) if we may be able to write them. And we can't. But we can *help* …
Clara:　　　　Reflect
Patricia:　　Yeah, we can do that.
Interviewer:　Is there any coordinator who writes [The Agreement]? Is it in the North region?

Patricia: In our region we don't. --- We do not. Because we are *not* a secretary to anyone. We are partners who cooperate!

The argument about exercising public authority is put forward, but the importance of "not being a secretary" took the argument one step further. Now, issues of the status hierarchy are brought into the discussion. The sensitivity of this issue was illustrated during a meeting at the social worker's office between Hedvig, the coordinator, a young girl, and her social secretary, Hanna. At the end of the meeting, Hedvig asked Hanna if she could revise The Agreement so that it was updated to the next meeting. Hanna said she could not undertake the revision of it. She had not made enough notes to do it. "Okay, but then there will be no plan written then," said Hedvig in a short tone of voice and began to put together her papers. Hanna said nothing. The underlying struggle was reflected in the tense silence and in the absence of nice collegial small talk ending the meeting. The young girl, their client, looked a bit lost when she followed the coordinator out of the office.

The vanishing act

Given the emphasis on the importance of The Agreement and the ensuing struggles, the last group interview with the coordinators was interesting. Very early on in the conversation, one of the coordinators summed up what the most important work "instrument" was, as follows:

Anna: The plans. It has nevertheless been our most important instrument.

Interviewer: Are you thinking of The Agreement?

Anna: I think of the implementation plans… which we used to call The Agreement at the beginning. (light dismissive laughter)

Interviewer: Have you changed names now? (surprised/confused tone of voice)

Anna: Well, it was like this: first we talked about The Agreement, then there were the treatment plans at the institutions.

Interviewer: That's right.

Anna: Then there are, in reality, implementation plans in the social service, which has become a concept for many in the social services, although it has existed before.

Interviewer: Is it called implementation plan when investigating child welfare?

Anna: It *is* implementation plans in *the law* (firm voice). That's what applies, see.

As there had been a strong struggle for The Agreement during the three-year project, the interviewer's confounded reaction is understandable: "Has it changed its name now?" The answer given was that The Agreement was something that existed *before*. The name belonged to the past, what was passé. In addition, it was "talked" about only as The Agreement, while the coordinator said that "in reality" it was implementation plans.

The interviewee "does expertise." She demonstrates her skills by teaching the interviewer the correct name. In addition, she claims that the implementation plans have "been around for a long time," just that everyone has not known about them. The coordinator not only teaches but also corrects the interviewer quite firmly. The interviewer's lightly confused response receives no understanding. When he asks if it is called "implementation plans," he is corrected: "It is implementation plans." The old Agreement is dismissed. The Agreement seems to have vanished into thin air.

This "vanishing act" touches on the emotional processes described in Chapter 3, *Seductive gatherings*, where members can work themselves up in meetings concerning issues or documents, but after some time, the contested issue seems to have evaporated.

Conclusion

Meetings and documents have a very close relationship. Meetings are often about producing documents, and documents usually require meetings to be established. We have discussed the spiraling administration as a result of meetings and documents generating each other. Some meetings are aimed directly at jointly formulating a document such as a policy, educational, or treatment plan. Other meetings are held to interpret guidelines, new directives, or laws.

There is an *Eigendynamik* in the taken-for-granted way of working through meetings—written directives are dealt with by having meetings or forming a new group or committee. The recurring audits that Power (1997) wrote about are often used as a "top-down" explanation for our accelerating administration. But there is also a responding practice that generates meetings and documents by the mere anticipation of such audits. That is a form of organization that not only presents the current state of affairs when evaluated but also whose representatives initiate meetings and collect documents in advance. Initiatives are thus taken from below, aimed at making the organization impressive for the outsider. We may interpret the project leader's happiness on how to proceed in the start of the project in this way: deciding on two administrative tools—being a chair during meetings and inventing a new document—might seem far-fetched in relation to helping the young people to a better future, but in terms of presenting the project to external organizations via new documents and brochures these items might have come in handy. It gave an image of a well-reflected orderly plan.

Our analyses of *Eigendynamik* have as the starting point the dynamic of order–disorder. The quest for order gives rise to demands for documents or meetings that clarify issues. We provided examples of how documents can solve problems pertaining to meeting forms, and how problems with documents can be solved through meetings. But the core of this chapter is devoted to a study of a youth project illustrating how conflicts about a document, The Agreement, may perpetuate via meetings and comparisons with other documents.

The Agreement succeeded paradoxically in relation to its name, creating disagreements and conflicts that were often unresolved. This particular document served as a symbolic object reflecting ownership of various documents, competence struggles, and the struggle within and between occupational categories over division of labor. These struggles were acted out in meetings and generated new meetings as various professionals wanted to discuss or criticize what this document would lead to in their particular context.

We argue that such conflicts may propel the administrative *Eigendynamik*, spinning around itself in a self-preserving fashion. When that spin is placed in settings in which ideas of rationality (order) and "everybody's involvement" (democratization) are strong, it turns into an expanding spiral. As we have seen above in the coordinators' clashes with staff from the social services and treatment staff at detention homes, ideas about what is rational may differ.

What we also saw in our case example was the coordinators' accusations of lack of effective leadership. In the next chapter, we look at how meetings offer their participants, especially chairs, a chance to dramatize administrative competence and how success in doing so can perpetuate interest in meetings and the administrative *Eigendynamik*.

Notes

1 An interesting but different lens on this relation can be read in Høybye-Mortensen's (2015) analyses of social workers and their artifacts, where she discusses how social workers talk about how they use different programs, questionnaires, and documents in their meetings with clients.
2 In Swedish: "Samordnarrollen inom vårdkedjeprojektet ungdom-MVG."

8 Dramatizing administrative skills

In Wilbert van Vree's (1999) study of the history of modern meetings in Western societies, he concludes that meeting behavior has undergone a process of professionalization from the 1930s. This process has also had ramifications for knowledge and experience of meetings in terms of social mobility: "As far as meeting behavior was concerned, competence and knowledge became essential ingredients for a successful career /---/ Whoever wishes to rise in present-day society has to climb the meeting ladder" (van Vree 1999:200-201). As we saw in the last chapter, even collaborators who disagreed with the idea of the document The Agreement still attended meetings to discuss it.

Indeed, in most organizations today, there is a moral expectation of a dedicated employee taking part in various workplace meetings. To behave properly during meetings is important, but so is attending them in the first place because doing so may make or break career opportunities. One's presence demonstrates commitment to an organization. In Schwartzman's (1989) study of an alternative health organization, many long meetings were held, and they often lasted until late in the evening, yet employees were expected to participate. The fact that the organization she studied was meeting-intense might partly be because of its activism and strong egalitarian culture. Such features recall Francesca Polletta's (2002) *Freedom is an endless meeting*, a study of social movements in America during the twentieth century which was characterized by their participatory democracy. These types of organizations, distinguished by a strong, democratic ideology, harbor members and employees who are expected to show great personal commitment.

The same expectation, however, is evident in Harry Wolcott's (2003) study of a principal in an American elementary school, which is not characterized by the same egalitarian ideals but is instead a fairly traditional institution. The principal insisted that the teachers take part in various meetings, also during evenings, and he himself attended many meetings that were not necessary from a formal point of view. Wolcott (2003) argues that in relation to the nexus of roles in the school context, meetings serve other purposes than the manifest and formal ones of negotiating and decision making:

DOI: 10.4324/9781003108436-8

First, they served to validate role—to give visible evidence of being engaged with the "problems and issues" of schooling. Secondly, and more importantly, they served to validate existing status hierarchies and to provide a continuing process for reviewing each person's position in those hierarchies.

(Wolcott 2003:122)

Not only is attending meetings important, but also important is how one behaves as a chair, a secretary, or an ordinary meeting member. Such knowledge is not mainly gained through formal training, as the social anthropologist Simone Abram (2017) has pointed out in the article *Learning to Meet*; instead, skills are acquired through learning by doing. From her study of council meetings in Norway, she concludes that both politicians and bureaucrats learn to be skilled meeting participants by attending meetings and observing others:

Participants in meetings learn to invoke the authority of the state through repeated practices of using role-names; referring to other meetings; choosing political rhetoric for symbolic effect; referring to statutes, regulations, shared knowledge, or norms. /---/ Such practices must be done with skill that is learned largely through participation, observation, and experience. The skills learned are constantly tested, since meetings are not always predictable. They could therefore be understood as classic social skills; without delving into detailed debates about social practice, it is useful to invoke the idea that social action is a kind of improvisation or extemporization building on learned patterns and categories applied in new ways.

(Abram 2017:87)

Abram gives one example of such a "learning occasion" from a council meeting in Norway:

After a little while, one of the deputies begins to discuss an issue with another member across the table. The mayor interrupts her, politely, saying that as she is a new deputy who hasn't attended council meetings before, perhaps she hasn't understood the procedure. He explains that she must always address her comments to the chair of the meeting [himself], and not talk directly to other members. That is how council meetings are run. She apologizes, a little flustered, and tries to repeat her comments to the mayor, somewhat deflated.

(Abram 2017:70)

We have observed meeting participants stumbling in a similar way in our studies, followed by polite guidance or correction by the more experienced attendees. Such informal learning also takes place in relation to paperwork.

Marte Mangset and Kristin Asdal (2019) write about the bureaucratic power of note-writing and how this is learned at work. They refer to how Weber, in his famous analysis of a bureaucratic way of organizing society, noted that not only were formal skills associated with bureaucracy but also a special kind of knowledge was: "*Dienstwissen*, forms of knowledge and skills stemming from the experience of service in itself" (Mangset and Asdal 2019:579). The authors observe, for instance, how bureaucracy directed upwards requires a high level of skills in note-writing and special kinds of writing skills according to the senior civil servants they interviewed at the ministries of finance in Britain, France, and Norway. A British interviewee said:

> The things that the team produces range from very simple kind of lines, to … take briefings for ministers, so that they understand the policy which is already set, so that they have the most effective lines or facts for communicating that policy properly. That's really simple stuff … to kind of explanatory notes, if the chancellor or another minister has asked a question about … let's say, about quantitative easing scores in the public finance statistics. Then we'll produce a two- or three-page note which explains what the concepts are and how it works. And then there's submissions which are policy advice, you know, ten pages, twelve pages. If it's getting beyond twelve pages, then you've probably written too much.
>
> (Mangset and Asdal 2019:579)

High skills in note-writing, as the civil servants learned in informal ways, can also be seen in less high-status occupations, as among ordinary staff at detention homes for young people. Some attendees, but not others, are tasked with writing the required diaries and journals that the organizations require. These were the people deemed competent in the art of written formulations (Wästerfors and Åkerström 2016).

When people are asked to describe the qualifications necessary to carry out a particular task, we can also discern a dramatization of such skills. The civil servant's explanation of how to write notes for ministers can be seen as a self-presentation of competence and know-how. This person will harbor the (inside) knowledge that the minister cannot handle more than twelve pages: "If it's getting beyond 12 pages, then you've probably written too much." Furthermore, ministers need simple kinds of lines, or two or three pages that explain the concepts and how it works. We can also discern it in the extract above from Abram's study of the council meeting in Norway, where the chair presents his knowledge and expertise through rebuking the wrongdoer.

Below we will dwell on the dramatization of professional and competent administrative management, especially focusing on meetings and the role of a competent chair. This analysis thus ties into Goffman's (1959) analysis of self-presentations and its expansion by later researchers. Catherine Kohler

Riessman (2002) has for instance, pointed out that we not only present ourselves with manners, poses, or choice of style but also with descriptions and stories.

Administrative skills can be portrayed in terms of being efficient, and artfully improvising when participating in and chairing meetings, as well as preparing and setting up future groups for meetings and governing their outcomes. To such skills we can add writing documents and reports and producing graphs and slide shows—activities that also become sought-after competences and consequently ingredients in self-perpetuating dramatizations, as we discussed in Chapter 6.

Below, we highlight how both skills during meetings and in arranging meetings are portrayed by participants who—we argue—can be expected to enjoy such descriptions and furthermore enjoy the collection of administrative experiences that gives material for such dramatized retellings.

Enacting the role of the chair

Interviews with managers, who often acted as chairs, make evident that they differentiate between meetings in which they are the chair and those that they have to attend as ordinary participants. We recall the university manager from Chapter 4 who said: "When you attend the large faculty meeting where the dean informs all the chairs from different departments, it becomes very much 'informing us' … rather boring, that's when you start looking at your emails, and so on."

On the other hand, being a chair is engaging: it demands orchestration and direction of the meeting and it demands attention. Moreover, the chairs might have a plan about what the meeting is to accomplish. Thus, in interviews, managers explain that when they are chairs, they are usually not bored even though they are "captive" in their meetings, in contrast to meetings that they do not chair. Being a chair can be involving, but it can also demand dramatizing and expressing the role. This may be done by the mere seating round the table, but it also can be done with props, such as a chairman's gavel that once was part of formal meetings. But documents, a particular folder, or a binder can also express the role. Below is a fieldnote written by an observer during his first day at a detention home, when he did not yet know the staff and the roles of the various meeting participants:

> Viktoria sits at one end of the table and seems to have some sort of leadership role: she is the one with the binder that says "risk assessment," and she soon starts to go through the behavior of the young people during the day. /---/ She often returns to the risk assessment binder and turns to me [the ethnographer] from time to time to emphasize things.

The seating and the sign vehicle (Goffman, 1959) consisting of "the binder" worked as clues for the conclusion that Viktoria must "have some kind of leading role," that is, acting as chair. Besides the seating and meeting props, chairmanship may also be discerned by manner. Let's continue with field-notes from a detention home. The field observation comes from a collegium that is held for a full day, and the first two extracts are from the morning:

> Niklas directs the meeting, this is noticeable not only in his placement, but also in his way of speaking, sometimes a little decidedly and instructively, and how he allocates speaking time. But at the same time, he often lets the staff talk and present their view of a scenario. Sometimes, he allocates speaking time, sometimes the participants speak freely. At times someone raises their hand.

> I note how Niklas checks with the staff several times: he asks questions and summarizes what has been said. In addition, he often laughs—more than anyone else in the room.

After lunch, the meeting starts again, and the participants make small talk and joke around, and Niklas takes control to commence "the real meeting" (Atkinson, Cuff, and Leer 1978):

> "Now we can't waffle anymore," says Niklas and turns to the points he mentioned to me earlier. He switches to the point of "reassuring surveillance" and becomes a bit more demanding in his tone. In the past, he has used humor several times, now he is more serious, he looks directly at the employees and is straight and clear when going through the information. Some things that have happened are not part of a "satisfactory surveillance," he notes, and exemplifies with the case where a boy departed as he went to a public restroom while on leave.

Niklas demonstrates his role as a chair in several ways, not only by his placement in the conference room but also by his manner. He talks "decidedly and instructively," and he directs who will be assigned speaking time. Furthermore, Niklas laughs a lot during the morning meeting (more than the others) but switches in the afternoon to a more serious and demanding tone. As Pamela Rogerson-Revell (2007) has shown, humor and laughter are often strategically used by managers, related to shifts from formal to informal style at meetings. Niklas illustrates this tendency: after initially embedding the meeting in an informal, light atmosphere, he can demand attention when he turns serious: both in tone and by looking directly at the others when reprimanding them by reminding of their responsibilities in controlling the young people in care. In this way, Niklas directs and dramatizes the stance that the present collective is supposed to take: being serious and realizing the importance of surveillance, the issue discussed.

Being efficient and creating order

A common critique of many meetings is that they are a waste of time because they are inefficient. This instrumental view of why meetings are held (e.g., "decision making," "information," "making plans," "formulating a policy") belongs to a common, rational view of meetings: meetings are supposed to be held to bring about a concrete outcome. In studies of various organizations, it is obvious that members may share such understandings, as in Francesca Bargiela and Sandra Harris's (1997) comparative study of one Italian and one British company, talk in meetings was sometimes contrasted with "action" (1997:5-6). In Gideon Kunda's (2006:153,185) *Engineering Culture,* an ethnography of a large American high-tech corporation where employees had to engage in some quite ideological meetings they contrasted these with work-group meetings that felt more "real."

This take is in line with what the interviewed managers described as important in our various studies: structure and efficiency, often contrasted with experiences of meetings as unstructured, "not leading anywhere," or "a waste of time" (cf. Thelander and Åkerström 2019). But the interviewees described various ways in which they ensured that the meeting time was not wasted, by ensuring that the time was used in an optimal way. Erik, for instance, who is a manager at a youth detention home, talked about the importance of meetings not turning into a nice "coffee break." When the interviewer asks how he conveys this expectation to the staff, he not only describes the technical way of doing this but also portrays himself as a competent chair of the meeting:

Interviewer: But how do you go about being a chair?
Erik: If you bring up something that's irrelevant. "Do we need to discuss that now?" "No, what is it that we should be discussing now?" That you constantly manage …
Interviewer: Mm, right. So you're rather controlling?
Erik: Very controlling. And above all listening closely. Now this conversation is heading somewhere else, it's heading towards the ski holidays. Then you have to bring it back and focus on what we are supposed to do.

Erik conveys an image of himself as skillful in leading meetings: he is concentrated and focused, "listening closely," and "very controlling." Angela, another manager, describes herself in similar terms when she states that she is "very structured" in relation to meetings. Both managers describe a specific *time-work,* efforts to control the sequence and allocation of everyday events and activities, a "micromanagement of one's own involvement with self and situation" (Flaherty 2011:11).

Another way of enforcing—and thereby also dramatizing—efficiency is to make sure there are "time endings," not only clock time starters. Angela continues: "I perceived it as a problem, that one can get summoned to a meeting at 13:00, but there is no mention of when it is finished." Apart from watching out so that people do not "float away," Angela describes her time-work as reminding the participants of the time limit of the meeting: "I usually start the meeting with: 'we have this and this time at our disposal.'"

Angela, like Erik, manages to convey not only concrete details about how to run a meeting but also her skills in steering them. She is not a time waster. Furthermore, she implicitly contrasts this self-presentation to those that are less skilled organizers, those that do not set a time for the ending of a meeting.

Administrative competence may also imply creating order through documents. A manager at a university, Robert, offers an implicit critique of others when talking about a committee consisting of himself and three research-oriented professors. He claims that the traditional seminar culture in academia means that people do not adhere to their roles of sticking to the agenda or writing protocols.

Robert: I notice that now when I'm in this committee, for example, and it has been this… it has a seminar take on it, so to speak, and it's great at times for you to be creative and so on, /---/ but meetings also requires a little something else, namely a few rules, a small agenda, a little memo notes (ironic tone). Like now when I was away this Friday as I was traveling [and couldn't participate in the meeting]. And sure enough: no one has written memo notes and so ….

Interviewer: But this committee is there … is there anyone who is, has that role to be a little governing and formal?

Robert: I've taken it upon myself to be the one to do this … say that "unfortunately I have to do a little … we have to write minutes" /---/ … this time I was not there and then there is no one else that says "I write the memo notes."

Robert depicts the intellectuals, those adhering to a "seminar culture," in a somewhat condescending way ("it's great at times for you to be creative and so on…"), and he is using irony as a way of criticizing the others in the committee when he points out that meetings also need "a little something" in terms of documentation. This work falls on his shoulders, implying that if he is absent, the order breaks down: "sure enough" no one has done the memo notes.

An often-repeated dictate in handbooks on how to hold meetings and in various assertions from employers is to come prepared to meetings. An equally important skill that can be underlined is one's capacity to improvise or organize meetings in a short time span. During an ethnographic study of a psychiatric hospital, the researcher followed different managers' workdays. One day, Stephen, a unit manager, had been to different meetings in the morning and returned to his office.

Stephen connects his laptop, says that he will show some images later during the meeting. He glances through his papers, says that he prepared for the meeting during the evening before and adds that that's the way it usually is. "You realize that 'oh, tomorrow it is APT meeting [the compulsory *arbetsplatsmöte*, workplace meeting],' and then you have to prepare something. But usually it works out anyway," he says with a smile, and I nod. He says that he believes that today's meeting will be rather short, but he also adds that according to his experience, such things are hard to predict. "Sometimes I think that, 'that item on the list will be difficult, it will take time.' No, actually it doesn't, but then there's another item that I thought would be easy and brief, but instead there's a lengthy discussion about that one. So, it is difficult to know," he says.

Stephen explains that preparations are not always thorough, but nevertheless "usually it works out anyway." He manages to present himself as savvy when it comes to meetings. The ATP (the workplace meeting) that he refers to is a meeting where all staff are invited, and organizations are required to hold them regularly—often once a month. Many managers have described that these are supposed to be open and interactive and involve issues concerning all personnel categories. These constraints, however, make them difficult: many issues are not seen as interesting for all and as involving only some categories. Stephen, however, recognizes his own ability to be able to collect some items to discuss, and images—PowerPoint slides—to use. He is also prepared to be unprepared—at times there are some items that you think will be easy and short "but instead there is a lengthy discussion." Furthermore, he is "doing expertise," as he is an experienced employee, even if not always very prepared: "It usually works out."

Mastering emotions

The modern meeting culture demands emotional discipline (van Vree, 1999). This means that anger, indignation, humiliation, or, for that matter, excessive excitement should not be revealed, or rather, should not be expressed too openly, only in appropriate forms.

In our interviews with managers, they tell quite a few stories about emotional states before, during, or after meetings. But with practice comes skill: after a while, one may learn how to hide emotions that are deemed inappropriate. One of the managers described how he could be nervous in larger contexts in the beginning of his career as a manager. He could be tense and have "a little irritation in the stomach and stuff like that," and:

> … it was hard to meet some people whom one knew one had a slight conflict with. I no longer experience that. I think I'm pretty good at arguing, I think I'm pretty good at … how should I say … both reflecting, stuff like that, and staying focused.

At other times, the chair may need to keep others' emotions at bay. During meetings, we could observe how a chair could do this with the help of invoking "going concerns" (Hughes, 1984) which originally referred to a whole institution as a concerted activity. Wästerfors (2011) expanded this concept to show how staff in a youth care setting could put an end to disputes with the help of everyday concerns, such as meals, lessons, breaks, or other mundane but concerted projects. In the context of meetings, "going concerns" can imply the different items on the agenda. In a team meeting with coordinators in a youth care project, the conversation touches on the sensitive issue of ethnicity:

> Coordinator Britt thinks that most of those involved in the youth care are not Swedes, which makes Mustafa [another coordinator] wonder what she means. Britt maintains that although they are Swedish citizens and many are born in Sweden, they are not Swedes and can't be because their parents are born abroad and keep up their own traditions. It's clear that Mustafa does not agree: "they can certainly be Swedish and want to live as Swedes." The other two coordinators also seem skeptical, and one of them says with a smile, "Keep in mind that we have a researcher here with us," thereby probably pointing out that stating that these young people are not Swedish cannot be "politically correct." The discussion is slightly edgy and charged until Per [who chairs the meeting] says that: "Now I think we should move on to the next point on the agenda."

When one of the coordinators points to the researcher and reminds the others that he is there, it can be seen as a way of jokingly breaking the tension. But pointing to the next item on the agenda—the meeting's going concern—put an effective brake on the interactants' involvement in the issue of the meaning of ethnicity. When the researcher brought up the incident with Per, he smiled and explained, "you have to know how to run a meeting, lots of sensitive stuff that we've had to deal with."

Meetings may be construed as an arena that is emotionally demanding. Several interviewed managers have explained how they may have difficulties sleeping before important meetings. Meetings are thus not only the boring events that they are commonly referred to but also where the "action" takes place for managers (See Goffman, 1967/1982 for an analysis of 'action'). They are events during which competence can be presented and challenges met. When the interviewer asks a university chair about difficult meetings, he explains that some do not have what it takes:

Manager: Yeah, but you have to dare to get into the shit, so—or what, Lennart Bergelin [a tennis coach] said that to Björn Borg [a famous tennis player], "get into the shit," like "keep at it," don't think so damn much but get in there! You must not think so much so that you don't dare. There are many who do, they pull out, they figure out beforehand what horrors can possibly happen and unfortunately they skip participating in meetings. It happened at times that I really wanted more of them to join, people have come to me and said that "I understand that you want me to join but I just can't take it" and then they've been sitting and thinking that it can be this way or, and "I don't like that, I don't want to be together with that and that person."

Then he describes his own stance:

Manager: Well, you have to have some of these meetings and then you're, like … you're really—it's like before an exam or whatever, you're really tense or like an actor who's entering the scene or, that's the way it is and… Sure there are nights you don't sleep, 'cause you know that at 10 tomorrow I have this meeting and it must not go to hell, it just has to work.

Interviewer: Yeah, I recognize this, some meetings make you really exhausted.

Manager: Right, really stealing a lot of energy, especially those that have, how to put it, yeah, either emotionally hot and /or a conflict that you try to solve /---/ [Meetings] who gave such tensions and these … brrrrr [expressing uncomfortable feelings] so huh, and sometimes it's like you can't even brrrrr because then you have to throw in a lunch, then it's a meeting again (laughter).

While others think about all of the "horrors" that can happen during a meeting, he himself has what it takes: he dares to "get into the shit." Even though his statement is focused on others' troubles and missing strength, a self-presentation is made through these contrasts. He ends this part of the interview by explaining that even if he lies awake the night before a crucial upcoming meeting, he *will* attend it, and furthermore, he is someone who does not give up. He has stamina. And after such a difficult meeting, the next meeting is just around the corner.

Contributing experiences and knowledge

One of the attractions of attending meetings may be the contribution in terms of the experience and knowledge an attendee can bring as a participant. We observed during all meetings how meeting members "came alive" when it was their turn to report, or if they felt that they had something to add on a subject being discussed. Such feelings of valuable participation may be dramatized in retold stories or descriptions and presented as a skill of being a manager. Some managers describe that the awareness of the importance of participants' feeling included made them engage in efforts to involve them. One of them, a manager at a detention home, explained when asked how he tried to govern meetings: "I like to delegate tasks to the staff, it makes them feel important, and then they perform better."

A strategy manager from a large city's planning council who has been involved in a meeting chain with managers from different city council departments can serve as an illustration of how managers tend to dramatize their own contributions when interviewed for our project. The group he belonged to was meant to organize the process of building new schools. This had turned out to be a long, tedious, and rather difficult journey with several low-key controversies and negotiations (Hall, Leppänen, and Åkerström 2019). The interviewee describes how the chair, Martin, who was responsible for this group, originally thought that the assignment would not be too difficult. But he came to realize "wow, there's a lot happening here."

> But I've been working on this for a long time so I see it as a good forum. So I see this as an opportunity to help Martin [the chair] with his job but also to go forward in the process. If we can finish this in a good way, it will be fine. And the more people that participate … we'll get all parties on board.

Even if the strategy manager did not appear very enthusiastic during the chain of meetings that we observed or contribute visible concrete solutions according to our fieldnotes, he retells his experiences by highlighting his contribution. Thus, being somewhat of a sounding-board is also a role that can be portrayed as valuable and a way of presenting oneself as a person with experiences and competence.

Manipulating meetings

Another meeting skill is the ability to manipulate meetings, which may occur in many ways. These strategies require some know-how that can be implied or emphasized in self-presentations. Here we present a couple of examples of this skill. The first concerns the importance the interviewee places on electing a chair and the interviewee's own role in this process. It is a civil servant who explains the process of choosing a university chancellor. The process involves a hearing with almost 100 persons, an assemblage of teachers, students, and technical-administrative staff.

Interviewee: When the congregation meets for the first time, there is no chairman. Then I've made sure that someone suggests a person who we think is a good choice. These are events with 90 people.

Interviewer: It can be unruly otherwise?

Interviewee: Yeah, it can be, it can just go to the dogs, catastrophic (laughter). It *has* to be manipulated (laughter). Otherwise, it can go either way. It's important who is chairing such a congregation. You never know how it goes. It's always palaver and disputes—It should be someone who is used to being a chair.

He can be assumed to anticipate the critique against such manipulation (selecting a chairman beforehand)—that it makes democracy but a masquerade—with the statement, "It *has* to be manipulated." As a civil servant, it may be part of his professionalism to assure that the meeting does not result in chaos or end up in no decisions with an ineffective chairperson. So there is no hesitation when he declares, "I've made sure that someone suggests a person who we think is a good choice." The "I've made sure" also points to his having quite a lot of power in influencing the outcome. He knows how to orchestrate such an event.

The way "to make sure" decisions go one's way is to learn how people in one's organization view various issues. One department chair thus talked about his strategy as "managing by walking around."

> If you take the board, for example, I knew that, here we have, here we have a question that we obviously don't agree on eh … so there so … I went around before (the meeting) and listened to what people said, I had about fifteen persons in the house that I could go and talk to /---/ if I noticed that, like this isn't sufficiently processed I tried to move the decision [to another board meeting] so that we would have time to talk about it.

A skilled meeting participant is also someone who has an ability to manipulate decisions during meetings. One such case was exemplified in an interview with a civil servant. When the interviewer asks about what ways a chair can be skilled, he answers:

> There [in the meeting] you can probably manipulate. If it is a controversial decision, it can be a bit risky to try to manipulate. I was present when such an issue came up, a controversial one. But at that meeting, when that issue came up, then the chair actually *began* by saying, "This is how I see it." A chair *never* does that. A chair says what he or she thinks last of all. That's what I've learned. But she clearly stated, this is what I think, like "and then you can think what you want." There were many who raised their eyebrows when she did that. It could've led to quite a bit of resistance. Now she didn't get it [resistance]—and maybe she knew it in advance. The proposal itself was bad.

We have mentioned how meeting participants are expected to follow norms in relating to meeting behavior (in relation to turn-taking in talk, disciplining emotions, etc.), but apparently meeting participants may deviate from these norms. In this case, the chair voices her opinion early on before the others have been given the chance to take a stand. In the interviewee's experience: "A chairman *never* does that." The narrator thus both presents his knowledge of suitable meeting behavior but also some admiration for the chair who knew when and how it would be beneficial for the organization to break a norm.

Arranging successful meetings

Another type of skill our managers implicitly dramatized was how they successfully organized groups or projects, arranged meetings or fixed meeting outcomes, and organized new types of meetings. Suggesting and organizing new groups or projects may entail not only the power to do so but also in many cases some sensitive talent in knowing whom to approach, when and how to approach them, and how to formulate one's ideas.

A case in point is the way the initiator presented the birth of a project on which border police and coast guards in countries around the Baltic Sea collaborated. As we followed this project, we asked the project leader how it came about. The project was thought up and driven by the head of a large Swedish regional police border organization. As the project leader, a high-ranking police officer, was involved in many projects and collaborations, he described how he strategically suggested his idea of a new project in small-talk when meeting relevant people. Such efforts may suggest some diplomatic skills:

> I meet the regional heads now and then, so I meet them and propagate. [I: Mmm] that's where I bring it up—I meet a lot of people, over time and plant some ideas with some and then we'll come back to it again and have a discussion, and I notice if you are interested. If they are not, then we can take it another turn and then maybe you can move on from the part you are interested in and take a meeting specifically on a specific cooperation issue.

He describes his way of maneuvering as using the opportunities presented at different events. In the quote above, he referred to how he would "plant ideas," and in the continuing interview, he talked about the importance of "sowing a small seed," "inquiring," and "propagate." And he explains that one cannot be too assertive and portrays himself as being diplomatically smart enough to wait for a better occasion to come back to talk about the issues the other party seems to be interested in.

The project was eventually financed and subsequently deemed a success by the participants (Yakhlef 2020). Therefore, the project leaders wanted to continue with yet another similar EU-based collaborative project. Europol, the former participating countries, and the highest level in the Swedish border police encouraged them to write a new proposal. In the meantime, the Swedish police had been reorganized, and now with the aura of success after the former winning project, many parties wanted to be involved.

This interest turns out to be cumbersome. Former and new department heads, as well as a whole new division, now want to "own" the new project.

"And then they have meetings, and then it was concluded that this can't be done in this way, but it has to be presented and discussed at the national operating council," says a member of the project team, who gets the assignment and tells how he went about it:

> … and then it goes back to me, I get to sit down and write a presentation PM, and then you have to present it and then it should go down … [in the organization]. See, projects are run by people, people who are passionate about it and have ambitions. Now I know this world, and I'm pretty stubborn and so on. And I can talk for myself, as you've understood. But, if you have, say John Doe out in the organization who is a little insecure but who may have a really good idea, he'll surely die slowly before those wheels have turned—but I know the people and where those I need to talk to are placed.

In both cases, the project initiators emphasized the need to talk to the right people to be able to go forward with their ideas. They interact during other formal meetings but also mention some communicative events that seem to be more of a one-to-one interaction. They also mentioned the importance of "a night out" to influence candidate project members and thus regretted the choice of a new top manager who was, as one of them explained "too much into jogging and a healthy lifestyle."

Both talked about diplomacy, even if not using this word. In the first case, the project leader mentions careful suggestions and hints, and in the second case, the interviewee emphasizes personal social knowledge, stubbornness, and endurance of bureaucratic realities. Common to both, however, is how their narratives demonstrate a competent self-image: they know how to work their way through their own and other "neighbor" organizations.

Coming up with ideas for new types of meetings may also contribute to the *Eigendynamik* because these new types of meetings may be a response to critique of meetings. Such critique was aired in the case of the collaborative project between border police from different EU countries (Åkerström, Wästerfors, and Yakhlef 2020). Collaboration seems to require meetings, but the officers involved in the project early on emphasized that they wanted to avoid "a lot of meetings" in line with an action-oriented police culture that celebrate physical toughness and the arrest of criminals. Still, the whole project was arranged in a string of meetings. When the project was evaluated, the police officers declared that the project was a success (despite all meetings). Why this sudden change of opinion? The researchers showed how the police officers successfully turned these meetings into "real police work" by removing them from the category of bureaucracy and its associations with formalities and rigidity. This was accomplished partly by omitting the word meeting: a weekly "operational action group meeting" was renamed "power weeks"—a "much less boring and sexier name" as one of the project leaders smugly explained. During these events more informal work and multi-tasking were encouraged to avoid formal overtones (Åkerström, Wästerfors, and Yakhlef 2020). Instead of skipping or enduring some meetings, managers may suggest new types of meetings.

One type of meeting innovation may be offered by new technology and seen as a time-saving effort. John, the head unit manager at a psychiatric unit, spoke many times during our fieldwork about yet another organization possibility, and quite enthusiastically, about the new forms of meetings that digital technology has made possible. At a meeting with other unit managers, one of them, Carol, complains about meeting time and suggests that review of the staffing should be possible to do in some other way, adding that she had to travel several miles for this meeting. John uses this complaint to argue for a new system, "Lync," which means that they can have virtual meetings and would save time:[1]

> John means that this contributes to much more efficient meetings because people don't have to travel all the way to the unit from nearby towns and cities to participate in the meeting. "It saves time and a meeting that would otherwise perhaps take an entire afternoon, can be done in an hour, because you don't have to travel," he says enthusiastically.

His enthusiasm is, however, not shared by all. Carol, who had complained about the time used in meetings, says that she can understand that, but the problem with things like Lync is that she uses it so infrequently. "And then you forget," she says, and the other unit managers nod in agreement. Both John and Carol lean on relevant knowledge when arguing: John in having found Lync and in acknowledging the need to save time, and Carol—with the others—in explaining implicitly that they have had experiences in trying out new systems: "you do it unfrequently, and then you forget." John's creative suggestion was not met with enthusiasm, and the issue of whether to adopt Lync or not was not resolved during this meeting. Lync was however used eventually, John was pleased and added that it did not only save time, it was a solution that was "environmentally friendly," too.

Managers can also demonstrate an ability to recognize the lack of appeal of meetings. Carl, a strategy manager in a large city council, declares his aversion to meetings: "basically, I think they are trying. From a need for freedom, I feel boxed in if my calendar is filled with meetings." As a response to the tediousness of conventional meetings, he explains that he has tested new types of meeting, in new places: "I have experimented with new methods and enjoy new contexts." It is not only because of his own emotional dissatisfaction but also that he believes he *has* to arrange more attractive meetings. The unit he manages has a very small budget, and moreover they have no legal authority.

> My only tool to somehow make an impression is that I and my colleagues and the products we deliver radiate confidence, wisdom, and

that you feel included /---/ [as] no one needs to care about what we do. So, when it comes to meetings, it's extremely important for us that we, the meetings we have and hold and arrange, and it can be all-day workshops and stuff, that we design them in such a way that people want to come.

When the interviewer asks when he realized that involving and including meetings were essential, he describes how the situation used to be. When he started, his colleagues in the council viewed his unit somewhat condescendingly, as small fry "doing something a bit unfeasible and unrealistic," and that they "had no muscles" But, he adds, with some triumph, "I don't hear that from anyone today." In this simple and short statement, he accomplishes a self-presentation as a successful manager who is using meetings creatively.

In the same way, he describes how he makes similar efforts for internal meetings. He allows discussions to go on and to be free and open:

> … so that it is not a one-way communication from the manager who, again, informs about this and this and that and such. Then there are such elements, too, but it must not dominate. Yeah but, making sure we have breaks, make sure you have small "hive discussions" [two and two], make sure something happens. Everything that doesn't happen in a standard, two-hour meeting, a little crowded room, too little air, no break …

Comparisons

As the classical sociologist Max Scheler noted, seeing oneself in relation to others is universal. A person "continually compares his own value with that of others … All jealousy, all ambition … are full of such comparisons" (Max Scheler 1992:122-23). In our data, we observed several instances of such comparisons in relation to administrative concerns, quite often used in dramatizing one's own skills.

Consider for instance, when a manager, a chair at a university department, discusses meetings, he starts by differentiating the social categories in academia: researchers, teachers, and administrators. During meetings, he then explains, it is especially the researchers who turn out to be less "meeting skilled":

> … they talk and talk and then like, let's continue talking next time. It's often those that complain the most even though they are the ones that contribute to that damn talk, which is not always productive and often beside the point.

Researchers seem in general to be a contrast category in relation to managers in meetings, typified as not being efficient meeting participants.

A strategy manager at a large city-planning council complains about boring meetings in the council getting worse when people from the university are involved:

> This type of two-hour meetings with the council administration, and when we meet with the university it is often three or four hours (laughter), where you feel that meetings, yeah a meeting is a bit like gas, it tends to fill the space it got.

Some interviewees also drew in others in implicit comparisons, but in opposite ways: some are better chairs than others. When one of the authors asks a highly placed civil servant how smart chairs can steer a meeting, he explains:

> The way they *are*. One of the most skilled is Axel Svensson (a former Minister). And also Marie Andersson (also a former Minister).[2] Very skilled. Clear and distinct: "Now we open the meeting." "Now we have this point on the agenda." Often you have an informal time for each question, each item, how long it may take. And they (the chairs) make sure that everyone who wants to make a statement does it. And in some cases, they make sure to ask if it's a controversial (issue), they simply ask to bring things up on the table. Then they round off when it gets close to … *Then* you make decisions and move on. It's an art to both push the meeting forward and to let everyone speak within a given time.

"It is an art to both push the meeting forward and to let everyone speak within a given time"—evidently there is more to the role of being a chair than following procedures, like opening a meeting, having an agenda, and so on. You have to make the meeting "go forward" and the ability to do that depends on who "they" are: their presence, their socially acknowledged character, and the way they act. The highly placed civil servant who is interviewed is obviously impressed about the chairs he mentions, both of whom can be expected to have a lot of experience in how to govern a meeting. In managing the tension between pushing the meeting forward (structure) and allowing everyone to speak (democratization), they skillfully manage the competing tensions in modern administration.

Being able to maneuver a meeting may not depend on the chair's meeting behavior only. One may also assume that "who they are," as emphasized by the interviewed civil servant, may mean "reputation." The chairs the interviewee above gave as examples may have had a certain *aura*, a sense of importance and mystique given in their being well known as former ministers, which meant that they met with less resistance than other chairs for the same board. The importance of a chair's reputation and standing may be assumed to hold for every organization.

Conclusion

In this chapter we have discussed the dramatization of professional and competent meeting management, such as in setting up meetings and choosing the relevant participants and suitable locations. We have especially emphasized how chairs may highlight their roles in their self-presentation or are highlighted as especially skilled by others. This analysis thus ties into Goffman's (1959) analysis of self-presentations. As Riessman (2002:701) argues in relation to such an analysis pertaining to narratives in interviews: "informants do not reveal an essential self as much as they perform a preferred one, selected from the multiplicity of selves or personas that individuals switch among as they go about their lives."

Being a chair offers opportunities for narrated competence displays, ranging from everything to applying experience and comfort with the process, controlling emotions and pace, doing meeting pre-work to manipulate outcomes, and adjusting meeting tactics and components to make them more interesting.

In making these efforts, meeting chairs not only dramatize their own skill and perform the role of "competent chair" but also ensure that meetings will continue, as they implicitly seek to leave little room for critique. Positive feedback for their competence and the effects of their skill in developing and running meetings mean that the administrative *Eigendynamik* will continue its self-perpetuating spiral. There will be more meetings.

As we see in the next chapter, the use of documentation to chronicle administration for the sake of transparency also ensures the ongoing spiral, one that may do more to muddy than to clarify processes. And in the give and take between meetings and documentation, this process also gives rise to more meetings.

Notes

1 The fieldwork was done before the COVID-19 epidemic, so time-waste was the only account given for this suggestion.
2 These are not their real names.

9 Muddy transparency

Documents are meant to bring order and clarity (even if their growth in numbers seems to indicate otherwise), as we have discussed in previous chapters. Transparency is another coveted ideal that documents are expected to bring about. The quest for transparency is a key issue in democratic institutions. In increasingly complex organizations (Bromley and Meyer 2015), infused with ideals emphasizing non-hierarchy, flatness, and transparency, there is a constant urge to identify and define who is doing what, what routines we can agree upon, and when and what mistakes are done. The importance of such activities is often indisputable. Clarity and transparency are overarching, self-legitimizing goals, and written guidelines and various reporting activities are often considered to be the key means to achieving such goals.

In this chapter, we focus on such self-reporting quality controls in the social services and in primary health care organizations. In particular, we home in on a specific tool used in such a process: the incident report. Generally speaking, this is the type of reporting that staff members are requested to do when something happens outside the prescribed routines and should be documented for the purpose of making improvements. Incident reporting is a practice presumed to limit individual mistakes by reducing as much as possible any informal dealings and individual solutions. It is often assumed that by minimizing informality and person dependency, professionality and efficiency will prevail.

Let us give an example from our own world within academia. In a recent information letter circulated at a Swedish university, all staff were informed of new routines for reporting cases to the caretaker department. No longer should the employees personally speak to the caretaker or janitor about even quite small issues. Instead, all problems or errors, no matter how minimal, should now be reported in a less personalized way, through a digital form. From the letter:

> Beginning in March 1, 2019, all reports about problems as well as questions to the caretaker must be made via a digital form.
> WHY DO WE MAKE THIS CHANGE?

DOI: 10.4324/9781003108436-9

We want to increase control over all problem reports, questions, and complaints that we receive. This is to avoid cases falling between cracks or being forgotten due to staff drop-out and new substitutes. The system provides both us and you control over all errors reported, with increased opportunities to obtain statistics and history.

In this example, there is an explicit account for the new routine. By making the staff file a digital report about a broken lamp in a bathroom or a printer that does not work, instead of calling or talking directly to the service personnel, the expectation is to reduce person dependency (as when someone is on sick leave and has to be replaced). The assumption is that there will be more control and that the organization will be more transparent through its statistics, paving the way for a systematic audit process. The ability to systematize the statistics is often an indisputable and taken-for-granted advantage to a rational, efficient organization.

In the analysis below, we focus on incident reports in the social services and primary health care. Such reports are mandatory and regulated by law.[1] They are part of the self-reporting quality control system that has increased dramatically in Swedish social services since the 1990s (Jacobsson and Martinell Barfoed 2019; Lindgren 2014). The incident reports in the social services and health care deal with a broad variety of deviations from normal routines that all professionals who interact with clients and patients observe during a workday. The reports may consist of a description of a mistake made by an employee, for instance omitting to hand out medicines to a patient, or any other incident that is perceived as "out of the ordinary" and considered to affect the well-being of the client or patient in a potentially negative way. Employees are encouraged to report their own mistakes or the mistakes of colleagues.

What constitutes a reportable problem or trouble is not always straightforward, however. The quote below is from a book based on a diary of the author's work in elder care. In this situation, two nurses have different opinions about whether an incident is worth a report or not.

> Nelly gets a bedsore, and the auxiliary nurse wants to write an incident report as Nelly has had to stay in bed too long, and has not been turned over in the bed, but the nurse stops it.—"I was perplexed. Should I report to the municipality myself? What is an incident? When can it be neglected?" (Bäsén 2003:165)

Staff may wrestle with issues around incident reports, as this short description of Nelly in a home for the elderly suggests. What exactly is to be regarded as a discrepancy from normal routines, and when and how should it be reported? The author of this diary, who is the third person present, is not clear about her own responsibility in this situation and what may induce a report or not.

In the following analysis, we aim to demonstrate how transparency efforts may obscure rather than achieve clarity, and how an administrative spiral is set in motion by such a process. In various workplaces, we have observed that once routines and guidelines for incident reporting are explained, new questions arise that in turn need to be clarified. A similar interpretative work was found in relation to the "SIPs" (documenting collaboration in the social services) discussed in Chapters 5 and 6.

Our analysis primarily details the interpretative work and the resulting self-propelling administrative dynamic that is set in motion by transparency efforts. In this chapter, we will demonstrate that this interplay between aspirations of transparency and interpretative work generates an expanding administrative practice of documentation and meeting activities. We will mainly use material concerning incident reporting in the primary health care and the social services for illustrating this interplay.

Undisputable quests for improvements

The previous literature on transparency has demonstrated that the quest for visibility inevitably conceals something (Strathern 2000). Embedded in the notion of transparency is the pursuit for accountability and trust, and as Marilyn Strathern (2000:310) points out: "As the term accountability implies, people want to know how to trust one another, to make their trust visible, while (knowing that) the very desire to do so points to the absence of trust." Trust has been discussed in relation to professional discretion, and critics of new public management have demonstrated how professional discretion is constrained by the quest for transparency (Garsten and Jacobsson 2016). Studies of the Swedish health care system have shown how the drive for transparency transforms an organizational field as it opens up for new actors (Blomgren 2007). Other studies have pointed out how mediating techniques and devices of visibility may not only create insight and clarity but also have ominous and ambiguous effects (Flyverbom 2016).

Although incident reports are common in many types of organizations, such as the custodian illustration mentioned previously, the effort to decrease person dependency and improve the audit system adds an extra moral layer to such activities. This moral dimension may intensify the interplay between the quest for transparency and more specific guidelines and routines on the one hand, and a dynamic interpretative work on the other hand. Care work in human services and health care provide an illustrative case of these dynamics.

Incident reporting was included in Swedish legislation through the regulation "Lex Sarah" in 1999 that stipulated that an employee in the social services has an obligation to report any misconduct or suspicions of misconduct within the organization (Jacobsson and Martinell Barfoed 2019). In our conversations and interviews with staff about incident reports in human services and health care organizations it is emphasized that the overall purpose of such reporting is to achieve a good standard of quality. To fulfill this goal, all mistakes and discrepancies concerning the treatment of a patient or client that are both within and beyond ordinary routines must be visible. It is only through such a practice, the reasoning goes, that the flow of activities and routines will run according to regulations. Hence, with the help of incident reports, the potential consequences of organizational problems or individual mistakes will be reduced.

Despite its relatively recent introduction, reporting as such appears to be taken for granted. None of the interviewees seem to have any doubt concerning the importance and value of a detailed description of discrepancies. In the interviews, when raising the theme of incident reporting, they often start with an embracing stance: reporting is a self-evident, indisputable, and morally recognized activity. A coordinator in home services describes the purpose of incident reporting:

> It is an illustration of risks. Either something has happened, and in such a case you have to make sure that it doesn't happen again, if possible. It is, I think… well, you have to display, sometimes the misconduct but above all the risks. So that you can prevent it.

Despite the lurking risks for clients, patients, and staff[2] if the job is not done properly or according to routines, the "risk" that seems to be at stake when incident reports are being discussed is the potential mismatch between actual incidents and the statistics. It is the reporting activity as such that is in focus. If the organization does not succeed in carefully monitoring the reporting, this failure may be discussed with regret, and staff may be reprimanded in staff meetings.

Providing good statistics is emphasized. If an organization underreports, that may have consequences, not the least financially as incident reporting is encouraged by economic incentives. The regional and local authorities have allocated "stimulation money" to increase the number of incident reports, an issue that our interviewees raised. It is, however, not seen as a solely positive form of stimulation, and some staff mention that overreporting occurs with a risk of encouraging quantity rather than quality.

As we will demonstrate, legislative and economic aspects are not the only factors that play a role in this intense documentation practice. There seems to be a more general discursive movement in the social services and health care around reporting. In a study of paperwork in the social services, the authors have identified a shift from a "discourse of complaints" to a "discourse of improvements" in relation to incident reports (Jacobsson and Martinell Barfoed 2019). This shift accompanies a more general change in orientations and attitudes towards incident reporting, from being a practice regarded as an expression of failure in the organization to one that proves how the organization is taking responsibility for the well-being of clients and constantly improving the routines. The quest for transparency has a specific orientation—aiming towards the betterment of the third party, the client. All forms of incidents reported by the staff should not, according to this discourse, be seen as failures but rather as opportunities for improvement and learning. This strong normative statement is repeatedly emphasized by employees and managers in our study:

> You know I've worked in health care for so long, when I started there wasn't any incident reporting, then it would've been really rough or wrong to write a discrepancy. Now it's seen more as an opportunity for improvement. But that wasn't the case before.

Despite strong normative orientations and an undisputable quest for improvements, with the betterment of the clients in sight, the path is not straightforward. Numbers and metrics may be used in unintended and less official ways (cf. Hjärpe 2020). As we will show, the less official uses of incident reports seem to be well known by staff and management alike, but they lurk under the surface. These possibilities are relatively unspoken, the kind of things that "everybody knows" but does not talk about—a form of public secret. This path away from transparency seems to evoke the urge to once again establish consensus and define, specify, and clarify, generating new ordering activities.

In the following analysis, we identify three types of activities that can be seen as expressions of the constant interplay between the quest for transparency and the interpretative work that results in expanding administrative effort. This effort is manifested in the production of more meetings and above all, more documenting. Two of these strategies operate in visualizing a workload, and the third aims to "keep your back free." These are examples in which the routine activity of reporting turns into something else, transforming the ideal of transparency into something more complex, ambiguous, and unspoken.

Reporting *en masse*

One unofficial purpose of this reporting practice is that it can be used as political pressure on management and politicians. For instance, interviewees have explained the use of reporting "en masse" as a strategy to make management aware of work overload among the workers. The goal is to demonstrate that the workers need more resources or else they cannot do their job properly, which will ultimately affect the client/patient. This tactic becomes a means of internal pressure in the organization and can also be used externally to put a pressure on politicians, described as a "fast track to decisions" by this social worker:

> These incident reports are discussed at the boards, the various political boards, and at that point they will probably just appear as numbers, but

still, it's something that quickly has a breakthrough in the whole system, and they're quickly getting through for decision. Then the politicians cannot say that "no we don't know about this" or "no we haven't got any indication that ...." It is just a fast track to decisions. And it's a system that everybody, just everybody, in the municipality is familiar with.

The "fast track to decisions" seems to work more effectively in extraordinary situations, however, such as when many refugees arrived in Europe in the year 2015. It was alarming when a vast number of refugee children arrived alone over a short period of time in Sweden, without parents or other caretakers. Below is an interview extract with two social workers, Maria and Lena, who describe their efforts in trying to take care of the troubling situation:

Maria: When we sat with all the refugee children and felt that we, but like "this, this we cannot solve," and we see that it will get on top of us, and that this can't last. And then, we really systematically, explicitly stated in the whole group, that now, now we write incidents on all this as well. Just feed it! [to the computer] And as you say, there could be 20–30 incidents per night. But we, in the end, we made them in lumps. But I… I think that has been very important. And I think we would not have had this extra staff /---/ if we had not been so very clear and consistent in this.

Interviewer: Was it a decision that you made together in the group, that is, "now we will…"

Maria: Yeah!

Lena: Yeah! --- I think it has been very positive because I think it [the strategy to report en masse] has led to a change.

In this case, incident reporting "in lumps" became a form of collective protest. In this specific example, the sheer numbers in such massive reporting had a direct effect, and the employees could see the immediate result of their actions in the form of extra staff. This situation, however, can be viewed as extraordinary and one that involves the clients directly. Others have said that they use the reporting as a strategic device, a form of protest or collective action, to signal precarious working conditions for the staff, such as too much workload. This strategic move is always at risk of being "discovered" or brought into the light. One example is the emphasis among some of the interviewees that hold a management position that although they need to improve the statistics, there must be "quality" in the reports. Staff should learn what is to be considered "real" stuff to report, not just "anything" or various things not in line with the overall purpose of the incident report:

And it has also happened, unfortunately, at times that when you've started to look at certain reports a little closer, it has turned out that there may not be much substance in them in relation to misconduct, but it may be more about problems in the staff group. /---/ That it becomes some kind of outlet, for frustration [but] that is something else.

These "other" purposes, such as staff issues, are not regarded as appropriate reasons for reporting. In sum, exaggerated reporting—for whatever reasons—seems to be an unofficial type of motive and application of the practice of filing incident reports. In those cases, the quest for transparency seems to have taken another, less clear, path. One result that is clear, however, is that this strategy accelerates the production of documents.

Picking the right words

Another means in the unofficial strategy of incident reporting is to specifically use and highlight particular value-loaded words or concepts in the reports. One example of this strategic use of language is to focus on "core values." The organization's "core values" being used in strategy plans and visions are conceptualized as both the fundamental values of the organization as well as "promises," such as always having "the best interest of the client" in focus. The conversation below shows that this strategy (picking the right words) requires a lot of skill and effort—but is still considered to be a "fast track to decisions." As this interviewee shows, getting things done through the bureaucratic machine is a struggle. In answering the interviewer's question about feedback on incident reports, this particular interviewee, Caroline, describes herself as an energetic person who seems to be proud of her own abilities to get things done:

Caroline: Well, the farther away, the worse is the feedback to those on the floor. So that it's also clearly individual. I'm someone who hunts down quite a lot. I'm not content with someone saying "we'll look at that" but I call and say "how did it go?"

Interviewer: How has it worked out, when you call and say something like that? (laughs)

Caroline: Well, it speeds up developments (laughs). No, but I, I, I'm so, I'm not sitting and waiting. But I, and I often rave, "these are the guidelines we've been given, that we should work according to, --- we can't keep to those, to our values that we should," and when you start talking about core values and norms and promises made, then most people usually listen. And realize "hey, hey, hey, yeah, mm, you're right about that." So that eh, some thick skin and not giving up. Hunt down people. That's how you get, good things happen!

"Some thick skin and not giving up. Hunt down people. That's how you get, good things happen!" indicates that the political strategies in such documentation practices are a very engaging task. But this is not enough. The smartness she portrays involves using the political rhetoric of core values and promises that most likely will capture the attention of the managers. The cleverness is also connected to a certain bureaucratic skill, a stubborn character as well as knowing how to use the right words.

Despite the bravado in declaring how one uses different strategies there seems to be a certain ambiguity in the system. On the one hand, the management and responsible authorities emphasize the importance of the incident report, but on the other hand, there seems to be an experience among staff that reporting is not always so popular. Hence, there might be different interpretations of how these reports should be used. Developing strategic skills for using the reports to make demands on management or politicians seems to be one outcome in this vivid interpretative work.

Hence, the "en masse" strategy—as well as the more elaborate form of using specific rhetorical devices, such as "core values" or simply sharp formulations—seems to be used strategically when the reporting practice serves as leverage to reach more than the official goal. These are examples of employees taking advantage of the system, in ways that were not meant to be, for the benefit of the client or the employees. It is, however, described as a work task in itself that seems to take a lot of time, emotional energy, and skills to achieve. But documentation tasks may also provide a sense of professional pride and integrity. Taking advantage of the system is a delicate balancing act, though. If it becomes too obvious or is itself made part of the system, then it might lose its status as an unofficial strategy.

Reporting "everything": keep your back free

Reporting en masse and using specific value-loaded concepts can be seen as forms of political strategy, with a clear orientation—from below and up in the organization, or towards external decision-makers. The following practice—reporting "everything"—does not have such a clear orientation. This strategy implies that the staff write extremely careful reports. Being meticulously transparent about all work tasks, reporting "everything," even minor incidents or discrepancies from ordinary routines, are sometimes explained as a means to "keep your back free." The interviewees emphasize that they really want to avoid being accused by colleagues, management, or the mass media of hiding information. This concern exists regardless of how trivial the act may seem at the time.

The reasons given for this practice—transparency driven to its extreme—may seem straightforward. These accounts, however, are often embedded in various types of complex explanations, with various moral accounts. Below is an illustration of how accounts of "keeping your back free" may be mentioned parenthetically and surrounded by several layers of explanations, demonstrating a complex moral negotiation around incident reporting:

> No, I rather think that it is a positive effect, or a positive input that one, that as [the colleague] says that now I must document extra, extra clearly so that our work can be visible, what we've actually done. That you –, partly a little to protect ourselves of course but also that you, that you actually get to find a solution that works for more people than just this little box that we're in. That you can't be that governed, that "we can't take them, we can't take them," but who should take care of these that don't fit into this small grid pattern? So that I probably think that it [the reporting] probably doesn't affect the work itself, the consequence can be that you feel that you've got your back free a bit, and then that you actually, that it becomes an extra-legal certainty for the client, and an added way to somehow try to help the client.

The interviewee above explains not only that one may want to protect oneself through being "extra extra clear" but also that reporting may contribute to "an extra-legal certainty for the client, and an added way to somehow try to help the client." Furthermore, she expresses a subtle critique of the bureaucratic form in incident reporting and the template itself: "That you can't be that governed, that 'we can't take them, we can't take them,' but who should take care of these that don't fit into this small grid pattern?" Not being "that governed," emphasizing personal responsibility and professional discretion, and reporting "extra extra clear" is thus a way to ensure that the individual incident, with individual clients, is properly responded to. The tendency to overreport, not because you are obligated to but because you are feeling a personal responsibility mixed with a way to save your back, is a tendency that we have seen in other forms of documentation, as well. In an interview with Anna, a school counselor, the issue of obligatory documentation is brought up.

Interviewer: You mentioned the duty to document, is that what's it called? You say you have a system now… but what does this duty to document really mean for you? But you have no duty…?

Anna: No, that's how I've interpreted it. We have no obligation to document, and then it shouldn't have an obligation to provide information later … but then again, it might be good to, say in a school inspection report, that it's in … there have been meetings with a counselor a number of times, and so on, not about what's been said, but that we've done it.

The practice of meticulous reporting seems to be an important reinforcing factor in incident reporting done in order to "keep your back free." Simultaneously, the interviewees stress that they are indeed taking personal responsibility for the client. The argument thus seems to be embedded in, and backed up by, various layers of moral motives because the very notion of "keeping your back free" is seemingly devoid of personal responsibility. It may even sound morally dubious to "save your own skin." Hence, the notion of "keeping your back free," in combination with stressing what is "the best for the client," can be interpreted as a means to resist the formalization and bureaucratization of responsibility associated with filling in the form while still stressing personal moral responsibility. The documentation practice of reporting "everything" might be a way of both embracing the administrative obligation to report and maintaining a sense of professional discretion. Hence, although meticulous reporting may seem like a clear path towards transparency, motives and practices are far more complex and ambiguous.

"It is not about blaming anyone, but ..."

In interviewees' accounts of taking responsibility for the client, we may discern a tension between a systemic perspective on the practice of incident reporting, as a form of collective learning, and an emphasis on individual responsibility. A coordinator in the home care service explains:

> What's good about it is that you investigate where in the (care) chain you have to make corrections, and whose task this is, whose responsibility. / --- / And that's why I think it's great with an incident reporting practice, 'cause it puts the responsibility back to the person who made the mistake. Like: "You! Re-do, do it right."

On the one hand, the possibility of tracking the chain of events, to see where exactly it failed is expressed as one of the great advantages of the system of incident reporting. On the other hand, when this systemic, rational perspective is put into practice, it seems to be transformed to an individual level: "whose task, whose responsibility /---/ "You! Re-do, do it right." At least, this is how it is expressed, and it seems to be a common interpretation.

Individualization carries the risk of turning incident reporting into a shaming process. Our interviewees related various stories about individual employees who have been "named and shamed" both within the organization and in the media for a mistake for which they were deemed responsible. Interviewees report on such incidents when the focus was on the accused employee and say that those individuals lacked collective support. There seems to be an ever-present anxiety among employees that this tendency to identify individuals will turn into a shaming process. A professional mistake may be personally detrimental, it is reported, and there is a constant anxiety of being the one who will be "named and shamed." Although the rhetoric says that mistakes are nothing to be ashamed of, there is a lurking disbelief, according to this social worker:

When you talk about it, you hear these words, that "it's not something you should be ashamed of, but it is important that we raise the issues," and all of that. But no one really believes this in their hearts. Everyone's a little scared and, and worried that it will happen to oneself. And let out a little sigh of relief when it does not happen to oneself, but it happens to someone else.

This perceived and articulated shaming risk is often counteracted within the organization. Several interviewees—particularly those with a management position—stress that the incident reporting should never be a means to name and shame. Rather, it should focus on the mistake being made on a professional basis, as a form of a learning process, so that it will not be repeated. They stress the importance of adopting a systemic perspective, not making it personal. A typical response is, "It is not about finding a scapegoat, it is all about having an overview, to make improvements in the organization."

Several of the managers stress the systemic perspective and emphasize how things have changed in the last few years. Incident reporting has "improved," which seems to imply that they have adopted more of a "systems thinking" and organizational perspective than previously. As we mentioned, there are tales of how it used to be and how it has now been improved:

You know, I've been working for so long in health care, when I started there was no incident reporting, at least not … unless there were some really bad mistakes, then you might have written something. Now it's viewed as a possibility for improvement. But that's not how it used to be.

Previously, manager interviewees say, there was a tendency to look at reporting as an exception, and the fear of naming and shaming was more prominent. As we have mentioned, this is in line with the shift from a discourse of complaints to a discourse of improvements, as identified by Jacobsson and Martinell Barfoed (2019). The discourse of improvements seems to be in tandem with a systemic perspective.

Reporting "everything" is a documentation practice that seems to be encouraged by a perceived tension in the organization. The simultaneous emphasis of systemic perspectives and identification of individual responsibility, reinforced by increasingly routinized reporting practices and the ideals of transparency, do not seem to create clarity for the individuals in the organization but rather trigger interpretative work. The inherent ambiguity in the quest for transparency has a self-reinforcing effect and initiates activities to define and clarify. A response to the insecurity evoked by incident reporting is the recognition that individual employees will have a hard time when identified as being responsible for an incident, and the quest for a support system for these individuals. This is how it is explained by a health care worker:

The purpose is not to punish anyone, but to improve the system. But then sometimes, there have been incidents when IVO [the Health and Social Care Inspectorate] came out and talked to the staff involved and /---/ the person who was the cause of the incident, she wasn't feeling very well. /---/ And everybody talks a lot about this, how do we take care of these people? /---/ it's such an enormous stress for these people. Nobody, ever, wants to cause any harm, unless you are a psychopath and most people are not! (laughter). Everybody wants to do their best. But sometimes things go wrong. And we need to talk about that. We have strategies for that, I think, and there are lots of articles and things written down about this, but we need to do more.

This quest for a support system requires new efforts, presumably new documents: "there are lots of articles and things written down." Incident reports generate new problems to talk about, strategies to be communicated to staff, new routines to be sorted out, and new items on the meeting agenda ("we need to talk about that").

Initiating an "ongoing discussion" and embodied routines

The employees describe as a dilemma the inherent tension between the risk of either being denounced or blamed by colleagues/or being the one blaming, and the urge to do what you are supposed to do according to the system. Hence, the documentation practice as such seems to encourage other types of administrative activities, such as meetings. The tensions and dilemmas identified seem to evoke the need to "initiate an ongoing discussion."

The following conversation shows how a manager for one care unit explains the need for a meeting called "the forum," which is a smaller meeting but with representatives from all categories of employees at the unit, in order to talk about the importance of incident reporting. She explains how they have to deal with the sensitive issue around such reporting, and how the forum meeting can "smooth" the issues.

I think that by discussing it in the forum, we de-dramatize it a bit. That everyone gets to see their piece of it all, comment, maybe defend themselves, and above all we can discuss how we should avoid that it happens again. So, since we started with this, with forums and so on, it has kind of softened it up a bit.

Another interviewee, Gunilla, further explains how the meeting, in her case the staff meeting, should work as a means to get incident reporting into the routines, as an embodied practice:

Gunilla: … we are quite new to how we register, we haven't got any good routines for it. Or yeah, we've got routines but we have

not started using — so it's not in our bones yet in a
natural way.

Interviewer: No, but how do you get it in your bones?

Gunilla: I don't remember what we have written, but that at regular
intervals we should take out statistics on it or the boss should
bring it up at the staff meeting with all the employees, that
now we have so and so many incidents, it's about these things,
what do we need to do for there to be changes in these, so, so.
That it should always be a lively discussion. And then I think
that the longer you do it, the more it becomes a natural part of
your work.

The documentation practice as such leads to another form of administrative
practice—the meeting—that confirms the importance of incident reporting
and turns it into an embodied routine.

Conclusion

In this chapter, we have shown how the quest for transparency and ordering
entails new and unintended practices that make the whole process far from
transparent. We have identified three types of activities that demonstrate
how incident reporting may serve other, less explicit purposes. The first two
documentation activities are organizationally strategic—reporting *en masse*,
so that politicians or managers are showered in incident reports, almost
drowned by them, and using specific value-loaded concepts to leave managers with no other choice but to consider the report.

The third activity highlights an inherent ambiguity in the organization. It is
the strategy of reporting "everything," an overly meticulous and detailed reporting, primarily used to "keep your back free," saving the individual employee
from being named and shamed as the sole person responsible for an incident.
This type of reporting is not only about saving one's own skin but also highlights
an ambiguous and complex understanding of systemic and formal responsibility
on one hand, and a more personal responsibility on the other hand.

Incident reporting goes back to the notions of trust and professional
discretion, which imply a certain level of individual judgment, based on
professional and personal experience. Thus, it is person-dependent. The
effort to reduce person dependency and the "human factor" calls into
question the professional integrity of human services- and health care
workers and is, although it aims to achieve a trustworthy system, an activity
of distrust. The contradictory outcome of such tension is the recurrent, "It is
not about blaming anyone, but we have to identify who is responsible."
Reporting "everything" becomes an emotional and moral response to such
inherent tension in the organization.

These various activities demonstrate that incident reporting is a type of
administrative activity with a self-generating quality. Meetings and ongoing

dialogues are initiated to clarify the meaning of the report, or following up on the reports, and the reporting practice itself is routinized as a recurrent item on meeting agendas. The overall goals with incident reporting are clarity and transparency, but in practice, the process feeds multiple interpretations, applications, and emotional and moral responses. All of which results in a spiral of administrative activities.

In this chapter, we looked at how a process targeting transparency, one that is intended in the end to be in the best interests of the client, can itself be an ambiguous, self-generating administration practice. In the next chapter, we look at another way that the attractions of administration can draw attention—and in this case, job roles—away from the client or patient. The allure of being able to educate one's colleagues in their professional practices, especially as a way to climb the professional ladder, can both perpetuate the administrative spiral and pull practitioners away from their original roles.

Notes

1 Patientsäkerhetslag 2010:659 se 1 kap https://www.vardhandboken.se/arbetssatt-och-ansvar/ansvar-och-regelverk/avvikelse--och-riskhantering/rapportera-och-anmala/
2 The risk for staff is mainly mentioned in our studies of detention homes and the psychiatric hospital when staff are encouraged to increase their incident reporting.

10 The devotion to teaching

In other chapters in this book, we have touched on the self-propelling mechanisms of administration relating to implementing new innovations or improving those already in existence. New digital systems are constantly upgraded or replaced, and professionals—teachers, social workers, doctors, and nurses—are required to fill in documents, digitally request vacation or reimbursement for travel costs, and carry out other administrative practices themselves. In a study of Canadian social workers, most employees needed four different systems for every interaction with a client (Baines 2006:203). Whereas most administrative tasks previously were carried out by administrative employees, they are now delegated to all staff (Agevall and Olofsson 2020; Forsell and Ivarsson Westerberg 2014). And when digital systems are introduced, upgraded, or replaced, the need for support is evident: new types of skills have to be learned, and they have to be continuously taught.

As university teachers, we have several times not only had to learn these systems but also encountered situations where administrators become engaged in teaching the systems rather than solving our digital problems. Our core tasks after all are to teach and do research, so the administrative work tasks arise randomly and are scattered over longer periods of time, which is why the lessons, once learned, are easily forgotten. Then we have to ask the administrators for help again and again, and they happily teach us again and again (instead of simply doing the task, for example, inserting the correct grades for students in the digital system from our reports).

This ambition to "teach the systems" seems to have a value of its own, apparently overriding the ambition to solve the administrative task. Furthermore, we discerned an ambition to spread the knowledge in relation to policy directions, security measures, and so on. In Chapter 6, *Beauty and boost*, we discussed the SIP document as an illustration of the administrative superstructure of manuals and instructions, the meta-documents of documentation that provide a form of learning material. In this chapter, we aim to further explore this teaching ambition and its driving forces, particularly how the teaching mode and practices may drive an administrative spiral.

DOI: 10.4324/9781003108436-10

Teaching the system as a "hidden" profession

New management ideologies, social work methods, and innovative practices in rehabilitation are constantly in flux in the human services sector. We can see a plethora of new management models and new systems being launched. These are models and systems that necessitate learning. This need in turn creates demands to teach staff about the right way to go about one's work. Doing so requires time to learn, methods to learn, places to learn, and possibly new meetings or meeting forms. Hence, it also requires teachers. We have identified some factors—structural as well as situational—that may reinforce the learning and teaching dynamic in the social services and health care organizations.

New digital support systems are illustrative examples of changes that are entailed by support services such as online mini-courses and instruction videos, personal service contacts, and specific educational services such as courses with consultants who specialize in teaching these new systems. There seems to be a whole supply chain of such services, constituting a market for technical support and educational services.

Apart from new markets for systems or management models, influential ideas and management philosophies may encourage a learning and teaching climate. The idea of the "learning organization" has been in vogue in management practice and theory for some decades. In a recently edited volume from the Oxford Handbook series, a number of scholars reflect on and discuss the value and future of both the theoretical concept and its practical value (Örtenblad 2019). The popular book by Peter Senge from 1990 entitled *The Fifth Discipline: The Art and Practice of the Learning Organization*, has sold 2 million copies and is often designated as the book that popularized and spread the concept.

Simply speaking, the idea of the learning organization is underpinned by ideals of holistic systems thinking, in which individual employees as well as the organization reflect and learn, ideally in a democratic and participatory way. According to Hoe (2019), the concept has not lost its value in research, although being criticized in various ways, but has changed geographical focus. It has now gained footholds primarily in Europe, the Middle East, and Asia, and less so in the USA where it originated, and by practitioners, it seems to be particularly popular in health care and educational organizations (Hoe 2019). We will not go further into the idea of the learning organization as such, but we can see traces of the idea, the precepts, and the discourse around the learning organization in the locations where we have conducted fieldwork. Vocabulary such as "learning" and "systems thinking" is prevalent, particularly among managers who are encouraged to reflect upon such matters in the interviews. Although we do acknowledge that such ideas take a foothold and influence everyday practices, we do not want to ascribe to them too much explanatory value. Rather, we see them as influential ideas that encourage and legitimate learning and teaching discourses and practices. They provide the cultural basis for an interactive practice where teaching, and the teaching mode, are attractive in themselves.

Furthermore, there are specific professional roles within the organization for which teaching is part of the job description. One example is the so-called compliance officer, which is a professional role designated to ensure that an organization is compliant with legal and ethical standards and that all staff follow the rules. In a textbook entitled *Essentials of Health Care Compliance* (Safian 2009:21), the role of the health care compliance officer is described in detail, and one of the most important tasks is "education and training of all appropriate staff members." Other professionals belong to the management bureaucrats described in Chapter 1, who do not have teaching in their job descriptions, but still involve themselves in such engagements. One example is communicators employed at universities in order to present popularized research to external audiences. Dissatisfied with the task of mostly writing press releases, some are now suggesting that they initiate courses in media training for researchers and university teachers. The communicators will thus teach researchers how to present their research appetizingly themselves.

As depicted previously, digitalization and the frequent launching of new systems, the educational and consultancy market, management philosophies, and new professions probably all play an important role in fostering a teaching mode and learning discourse. However, we do not think that these factors solely explain the prevalence of teaching activities and the teaching ambitions of organizations today. In particular, they may not explain the teaching engagement we have observed and the apparent attraction of engaging in such activities. In contrast to the designated teaching roles of consultants and specific new administrative professions, what we have observed is a type of teaching that is informal and often self-imposed. What we find particularly interesting is the informal teaching ambitions among staff at all levels in the organization whose formal role descriptions do not include teaching.

Hence, informal teaching appears as a "hidden" profession in the organization, with an attraction and value of its own. Although teaching may be a hidden profession, its value is often widely recognized and taken for granted in the organization. Carving out new meeting spaces and times for such activities is, as it seems from our study, generally not questioned and, in keeping with the administrative *Eigendynamik*, seems to have a self-reinforcing quality.

Interaction and dialogue as the ideal pedagogic form

One of the attractions of both teaching and learning situations seems to be their interactive and participative form. New models, new systems, and new routines need to be "anchored" in the organization, according to democratic ideals. It is often assumed that if this anchoring process is supposed to be effective, it is never enough just to "inform" the staff; the staff themselves must be turned into better administrators. Participative dialogue, in inter-action, and meetings seem to be regarded as a superior form of sharing information in a democratic institution, rather than one-way communica-tion. Overall, the interactive and participative forms seem to be taken for granted in the many scheduled workplace meetings we have observed. This acceptance is in line with what we have previously noted about democratic ideals as one explanation of the accelerating administrative tendency in contemporary societies, specifically in relation to what van Vree (2011) calls "meetingization."

The following quote is from a chair, a manager at a university depart-ment, who ponders the meaning of meetings when faced with a seemingly naive question by the interviewer:

The interviewer:	Why… do you have meetings?
The Chair:	(hint of laughter) Yeah, well … I guess it's for … to inform … to get … discuss, get a dialogue going, not only information, 'cause that can get done by… well … email or something. /I: Mmmmm/ But … that there will be an interaction around … around what would otherwise have only been information.
Interviewer:	Right.
The Chair:	So that things should be based on community … I can imagine.

The chair is evidently taken aback by the question about meetings: They are common and routine, but why do we have them? He is not alone in this insecurity; the meaning of meetings is now ambiguous and the meeting-landscape has evolved. It is not as it used to be when meetings were scenes where negotiations occurred and decisions were made (Hall, Leppänen, and Åkerström 2019). After some clear hesitations, he finally comes to the conclusion: they exist so that the people in the organization can reach an understanding together.

Educational situations, such as teaching new management models, are often designed to be particularly interactive because they also are anchored in pedagogic philosophies. We mentioned in Chapter 2 that the social anthropologist Renita Thedvall studied an example of a new management ideal in preschools, the Lean model (2019). The preschools in her sample had decided to organize themselves according to this model to become more efficient. As we noted, the model was imported from the car-making in-dustry and is meant to create a more efficient production chain. The human services have borrowed concepts from it, including teamwork and short daily meetings involving gatherings in front of a whiteboard to visualize goals and problems. To initiate this new model, the staff at the preschool had to attend a Lean course training:

> We were seated at tables for four, where a flipchart-sized paper lay. Lean consultant Karin, who was giving the course, pointed to the large sheet of paper and explained that it was supposed to typify Lean's problem-solving document, which is known merely by its paper size, A3. The flipchart-sized paper represented a chart that featured nine labeled cells.
>
> (Thedvall 2019:122)

The cells contain headings such as "problems" and "action plan." In this case, a consultant led the course, and the pedagogic form was interactive. Participants were divided into small groups, working with the material, discussing, and presenting. This course was obligatory for the preschool staff, as are many consultant-led courses.

At times, staff may show some resistance to the way Lean is set up, with whiteboards and daily evaluation meetings (Hjärpe 2019; Thedvall 2019). But some may find attractions in the new ways. Consider, for instance, one of the first Lean meetings at the preschool. Melissa, the preschool head, and Mira, the Lean coach, stand and the teachers sit down around a table. Melissa explains that they all have to stand up to stay alert. She then turns to the whiteboard and goes through all of the staff, asking them questions about how they evaluated one of the workdays (they do this by filling in red, yellow, or green dots). One of the staff, Caroline, is not able to explain why she has chosen a green dot.

> Melissa left Caroline and turned to Silva: "And then we have Silva; you also had a green dot." Silva responded that she had been to a Lean board meeting at Ladybug Preschool (part of the same preschool unit) and thought it was extremely interesting. She realized that they could do many things with the Lean board. She finished by saying that she would like to go to their meetings one more time to get more inspiration.
>
> (Thedvall 2019:97)

Her comment indicates an interest not only in attending one more meeting (rather than working with the children) but also to do so "to get more inspiration," pointing to an interest in learning more. Furthermore, the courses are often a getaway from everyday routines, sometimes held outside the workplace, often with lunch and coffee breaks included. Courses may thus have an attraction on their own because they interrupt the everyday workflow and provide an out-of-the-ordinary event.

Administrative pedagogy embedded in routines

In the preceding chapter on incident reporting, we demonstrated how the human care organizations emphasize and reinforce a discourse of improvement. Incident reporting has "become better," staff have "learned" how to write reports, and meetings are held to teach the staff to write reports with quality, not just quantity. As with specific courses, new meetings are held in order to initiate learning. But already existing administrative meetings also may turn into learning occasions. The following observation is from a staff meeting at a psychiatric unit, where the chair makes a comment about these incident reports:

> "But wait, didn't we skip item number five?" someone says, looking in his papers. The chair looks in his papers, too, and says, "Well, that was the thing about having internal training at certain meetings." "Yeah, okay," the first person says.

The chair continues and talks about incident reports, which seems to have become a routine item (item five) on the meeting agenda. Administrative meetings may turn into educational occasions. In that mode, the educational dimension becomes embedded in the organizational routines. Staff meetings are not only occasions for sharing information but also are transformed into learning sessions. In this instance, the chair himself (in his capacity as a manager) has an articulated responsibility to give feedback on the reports, something he thinks could be improved:

> "Incident reports," the chair then says, "there are no new ones written since the last APT [staff meeting] meeting. We are still waiting for the door to the medicine room to be repaired," he says (apparently some kind of awkward lock). "There are also two Lex Maria cases [incidents required to be reported by law] to be investigated," he says. Nobody asks anything about this. I [the researcher] get the impression that these are already familiar to the staff. The chair continues and develops his reasoning around the reports. He also says that they may wonder what really happens to the reports that are written. He says he thinks they can improve the following up and give clear feedback, and this is something that is his responsibility to give feedback on the discrepancies that come in.

The feedback on this form of documentation practice is regarded as important, so that the staff can learn how to report properly. As we discussed in Chapter 9 on incident reporting, the former discourse of complaints that previously dominated staff talk about this required reporting practice has now turned into a discourse of improvement. Improvement implies learning, including feedback and an ongoing discussion about how to make things better.

This organization also has a specific "patient safety group" that follows up the incident reports. There seems to be a consensus in the meeting that this is important and even that it "is about time" that the patient safety group is now up and running to deal with those reports. This documentation practice also seems to initiate the need to have specific courses. The chair brings it up:

The chair says that the reports are also followed up at the clinic. "It was a meeting in the patient safety group on 18/11, and there they look over the reports that come in," he says. According to him, the work in this group has halted for a while, he says that it has gone "a little up and down" with this group, but that it's running now. "Yeah, that's about time," someone says at the table. The chair nods and says that there have been a lot of reports at the clinic that concern threats and violence and that this is something we now want to review. He takes a document in his hand and reads that it's, among other things, about training staff in "treatment with security thinking." The participant sitting at the table nods and there is no further discussion about the incident reports. The chair says: "Anyone who has anything more to bring up?" People shake their heads, there doesn't seem to be anything else. "Then, in conclusion, we'll take a look at the new Patient Act," he says and starts the projector for the slide show presentation.

Hence, it is not only incident reporting that has become an integral practice in the organization but also the practice of following up and providing feedback on the reports. This extension sometimes requires new working groups, as in this case, with new meetings, even new courses, and possibly new documents. Chairs of the meetings, who are often managers, adopt a teaching role, making sure that the staff are not merely informed but that they also learn.

This learning and teaching dimension, apart from specific courses, seems to be embedded in the organizational routines and is not always visible because it is a type of ongoing teaching and learning informally adopted by certain staff. In a study of the practice of bureaucratic note-taking among civil servants in British, French, and Norwegian ministries of finance, it was clear that the skills of these high-level bureaucrats are to a large degree acquired during many years of service to politicians. An explicit part of their everyday work is to train new bureaucrats, lower in the hierarchy, repeatedly giving them feedback on the art of note-taking (Mangset and Asdal 2019). Interestingly, it is not the professional knowledge and formal educational training as civil servants that seem to be crucial in making a career and being skilled at work, but the generic skills in writing clear and to-the-point notes. Teaching and learning this specific administrative skill are thus crucial to a successful career.

The teaching ambitions as well as the generic skills of note-taking are in this mode "hidden" because they are not overtly acknowledged as part of the professional role, although "everybody knows" that this is an important skill. These teaching and learning practices also require specific time and space for feedback—editing the fieldnotes, giving feedback, and talking about how to improve one's note-taking skills seem to occupy a substantial part of the working time.

Devoted teachers

Once organizations decide on a management model or new digital systems to implement, new opportunities arise in terms of volunteering to teach. Who are these teachers, and why do they adopt this role? It is not uncommon that it is staff with some form of administrative position as part of their formal job description, although this is not always the case. Social workers, homecare workers, administrators, workers caring for the elderly and disabled, and preschool teachers are examples of employees who chose to become "Lean coaches" in the municipality that Thedvall studied (2019:93). In the case of the preschool, this meant that one school lost a trained coworker because the new task—teaching one's colleagues—seemed more alluring.

Critics of the administration society have pointed to new forms of professional boundary crossings in professional organizations. A tendency today is the de-professionalization of certain professions (since they need to do administrative tasks) and re-professionalization of former secretarial roles (Forsell and Ivarsson Westerberg 2014). Administrators today generally have higher academic degrees than previously, and new job titles have emerged (Agevall and Olofsson 2020).

The general tendency of the professionalization of administrative staff is sometimes combined with an upgrading struggle and an effort to deconstruct prevailing hierarchies. Höglund and Armelius (2003) showed, for instance, that administrators in academia are not satisfied with low-level administrative tasks. Such motives might underlie the inclination to teach faculty about digital systems rather than simply taking care of the bills and tickets that have to be fed into these systems. In the same report, the interview data show that this type of resentment over low-skilled work is not uncommon. This resentment discourse on the one hand centers on being disrespected and unappreciated and on the other hand involves claims of actually being very competent. Against such a background, there may be a certain satisfaction, based on resentment, in the power given by the audit society. A report edited by researchers Ivarsson Westerberg and Jacobsson (2013:41) relates statements from "witness panelists" (high civil servants and a journalist) about the audit society. This "scorned-delight theory" was suggested by the journalist Maciej Zaremba: "In the audit society, people with less education can scrutinize and haul over the coals the highly educated specialists/experts who cannot defend themselves."

New job titles among administrators, hierarchical repositioning, and resentment discourses may be some explanations for why self-imposed teachers see new fertile ground in teaching, perhaps viewing this instructional dimension as part of a new status and professional role. However, structural changes in the professional ecosystem may not be the only explanations, and specific situations also could encourage and evoke a new professional status.

The following observation is from a large event organized by different border police organizations in the collaborative project "Turnstone." The assistant Mona has the most subordinate position in this large-scale meeting, but her assignment is important: she is the one to keep all of the high-status managers from the various Baltic police authorities in order. After a successful application for funding from EU, they are now gathered in a meeting to start the project:

> After the introduction, Mona, who was mainly in charge of issues of funding and organizing events, described the extensive process of formalizing the project and of writing the project application. She then presented the financial plan, the allocated funding for each activity, and explained the activity list (from the EU application) --- Niklas emphasized twice that it was really important to follow the rules, and Mona added that all participants had to remember to send her their tickets and boarding cards after traveling to project events. Providing enough documentation of the project was very important as the initiators were required to write reports about the project activities. "It is easy to avoid mistakes," Mona said, by setting up routines, having follow-up meetings, carefully reading instructions, and taking the time to write reports on the meetings.... She clarified that impact in this context meant outlining positive outcomes of the project. One officer asked whether there were any report templates that could be used, and Mona promised to send these to each officer responsible for documentation.
>
> (Yakhlef 2018:102-104)

In this interorganizational network, Mona becomes the front-figure at the event, the one who has the overview and knows the administrative system. She becomes the teacher in the class, a role that emerged and became manifested in the meeting. In this case, it was the large-scale interorganizational meeting, the event, that induced a teaching role. As Andersson Cederholm and Hall (2019) pointed out in a study of interorganizational business events, some of these network-based social gatherings are often explicitly anti-hierarchical, with an inclusive vocabulary. A project secretary who doesn't have organizational authority in the "ordinary" work situation may gain situational authority in these types of meetings. This authority may safeguard the egalitarian network culture even more than if some of the managers of these organizations were to take this kind of role.

The previous example demonstrates a status subversion when administrators take a managing and teaching role. It also demonstrates how the social situation of the meeting may facilitate such a role. However, staff who are lower in the hierarchy are not the only ones who may gain status with a teaching role. There are possibilities for new administrative roles at the same level in the organization, and former social workers, nurses, and university teachers, for example, may see the possibilities of alternative career paths as administrators. For instance, since evaluations and control have become more important in contemporary social welfare offices, there is now a plethora of new positions. New titles in these offices include quality controllers, strategists, development leaders, planning secretaries, and methods developers. These are often social workers who have left their traditional occupation (Hjärpe 2019:165), who might be prone to taking on "teaching roles" in relation to other staff.

These teaching ambitions can be "hidden" and situational, as we mentioned previously, not even part of specific new professional roles. Many social workers, nurses, or teachers take on this informal teaching role in various workplace meetings. Let's return to a meeting discussed in Chapter 3, where Olle talks about the importance of incident reports. He is a school teacher at a detention home, but also has an assignment as the facility's safety ombudsman. At a staff meeting he is asked to report on his work in his latter role:

> In his capacity as a school teacher, Olle normally participates in the informal, joking atmosphere that is common in the meetings. But when he is now reporting in the role of a "safety ombudsman," his voice becomes very serious. He emphasizes the importance of reporting ALL incidents. This is not the case at the moment, he continues with a somewhat lecturing tone of voice. Everything has to be reported. The atmosphere in the meeting turns serious, and all seem to agree that this is very important. Olle becomes a stern teacher, reprimanding his colleagues about the importance in filling in incident reports.

We have seen several situations similar to this in our observations. These are situations where one or a few colleagues together are not merely informing but also teaching their fellow colleagues about administrative routines, documents, or systems. They temporarily step out of their ordinary roles: they become teachers, and their colleagues become students.

Conclusion

In this chapter, we focused on the ambition and attraction of teaching colleagues about administrative matters. These matters could involve new systems, new routines, or new policies. We have outlined some factors that probably play important roles in this teaching and learning culture, such as the ongoing launching of new digital systems and an accompanying educational market with a supply of courses, popular management philosophies such as "the learning organization," and new administrative professional roles that include teaching. We also suggest that these factors do not solely explain the attraction and ambition to teach. These opportunities offer an opening for the ambitious, forming an administrative pedagogy that seemingly overrides the necessity to have the tasks done. For administrators, the teaching role may have a status-enhancing effect. For other professions, it may simply be appealing to step outside the ordinary work role and be absorbed by a "teaching situation."

The administrative pedagogy with its teachers and students both legitimizes and expands administrative practices. As we have seen, some ordinary staff meetings turn into educational occasions, and it may be difficult to separate a teaching and learning occasion from other meetings. The educational dimension seems to be embedded in organizational routines, which create new motives for having staff meetings or to write, rewrite, or update various documents.

Certain staff members are sometimes selected to participate in a course to teach the rest of the staff, or it may just be taken for granted that the new knowledge acquired will be spread within the organization. Furthermore, the teacher/student role has an inherent self-generating quality because the student may eventually take the role of a teacher. Apart from cultural and structural dimensions, the interactive dynamics of the meeting situation as such and the preparations for meetings may turn staff members into informal teachers.

In this way, administrative pedagogy has a diffusional character, and we have depicted administrative teaching as a "hidden" task of a profession. Staff from all levels seem to be engaged in teaching and thus form a hidden faculty of devoted teachers. The teaching ambition does not seem to be reserved to administrative staff, although it may be particularly attractive to those who could see the teaching role as a status enhancement. Managers, for instance, seem to take a teaching role, as it is expected that they have pedagogic, interactive meetings and provide useful feedback to encourage learning. In this way, all staff are students, and they are all potential teachers.

In the final chapter of this book, we examine how executing these hidden roles and honoring the formality and intent of meetings and related documentation involves a certain morality. We take this expectation of morality, along with the human qualities of emotion and anticipating "magic," as a frame for looking back at the main themes of this book.

11 Magic, emotions, and morality

Contemporary societies have seen an ever-expanding administrative involvement. More and more people have to do paperwork in accounting for their job tasks, and new social categories are drawn into an increasing meeting circus, i.e., what van Vree refers to as a *meetingization of society* (2011). Police officers, doctors, social workers, and teachers now grumble about time-waste during meetings with other professionals and having to spend time on documenting their work instead of actually attending to their core tasks (e.g., Abramovitz 2005; Baines 2006; Erickson et al. 2017; Forssell and Ivarsson Westerberg 2014).

In our introduction, we referred to common "top-down" explanations of this administrative expansion, such as new ways of governing, democratization, collaboration, changing administrative occupations, and digitalization. In this book, as a complementary way of explaining the expanding administration tendency in contemporary society, we have supplemented top-down explanations with a new focus on the inner dynamics of administrative efforts: the everyday attractions and contingencies that keep people's appetite for administration alive. People are not only captives in meetings and by documents; these administrative tasks may also be captivating.

Our argument is that despite widespread complaints about too many meetings and too much paperwork, the process of doing administrative work contains hidden attractions, enticements, and entrapments that contribute to its expansion. We have tried to illustrate and tease out the self-propelling dynamics born out of initiatives from below. Via several ethnographic studies, mainly from the human services sector but also from academia and elsewhere, we have illustrated various ways in which meetings and documents can be magically enchanting and aesthetically appealing in everyday working life.

But administrative tasks are also surrounded by morality and emotions. As the anthropologist Michael Herzfeld (1992) points out, a commonly held assumption of modernity is that its bureaucracy is a symbol of rational government; he argues instead for a symbolic analysis of bureaucracy. People often routinely criticize bureaucracy but still embrace the morality and idea of rational administration, just as anticlericalism often coexists with deep religiosity.

DOI: 10.4324/9781003108436-11

The morality of meetings and paperwork

We have seen this implicit cherishing of bureaucracy in the irritation towards people who do not obey bureaucratic rules in documenting various work tasks or towards those who leave meetings early. Such irritation illustrates both the morals and the associated emotions. Meeting morals demand that you honor the gathering, and only the most exigent circumstances are allowed to disrupt it. At a detention home, we witnessed how it took an escalation of conflict into a violent incident for staff to pause a meeting; in all other circumstances, the meeting form was highly respected and carried on. Meetings seem to have a magnetic quality in workplaces, and the principles of meeting inclusiveness are highly regarded in the human services organizations we have studied. "I have a meeting" is often viewed as a legitimate excuse for not being available to perform other tasks, an honored account for being occupied and temporarily unavailable. In a hierarchy of work tasks and routines, meetings in general seem to be a top priority. Not going to meetings, or sneaking out too early from a meeting, are practices surrounded by different forms of excuses and justifications.

Apart from rule-based requirements, there also seems to be an attraction in the documentation practice related to what can be called a "moral ordering practice." The moral ordering is partly related to legitimacy and the controlling gaze of the third party—a higher authority—and partly related to an emotional satisfaction in "having all papers in order," "it feels so good to be able to check it off," illustrating how such efforts may represent an experience of professional competence and morals. Despite the affective neutrality that supposedly characterizes the bureaucracy, or as Weber (1978:975) summed it up, "sine ira ac studio"—without hatred or passion—we have found strong moral commitment and emotional expressions in relation to bureaucratic tasks.

And using time for paperwork may also have other moral advantages. That is the case at least according to Tiffany Taylor (2013:24), who claimed that caseworkers in a welfare-to-work program did more paperwork than interacting with clients. They prided themselves in treating people fairly, "to them, treating everyone the same, in terms of paperwork, meant being fair." Such a perspective can be seen as a cornerstone in the bureaucracy that we tend to cherish: obeying rules regardless to whom they apply (Herzfeld 1992).

Emotions and magic

Morality and emotions play out in observable ways when studying meeting and documenting practices, but the aspect of magic is also evident. The document itself opens doors, so to speak, both to professionals and their clients in the human services sector.[1] Some documents acquire a totemic status. In the field of human services work, the magical qualities of documents are also socially invoked in paperwork that seems to produce what is sought after—order, collaboration, quality, and more—according to the formula "like produces like" (Mauss 2001). If a nursing home can present the requested plans and documents, they are likely to be assessed as an esteemed establishment that provides "quality care." If they cannot, they run the risk of a lower score in quality measurements. To have a care plan in its documentary form equates to "having" quality (Jacobsson and Martinell Barfoed 2019).

A sense of order

In a very basic and general sense, documents and meetings create a sense of order. Society and its institutions and organizations are constantly changing. Human services staff encounter new demands, rehabilitation models, and policies, and they meet new clients with messy and multifaceted lives and new coworkers with personal working styles and habits. Well-established routines and the taken-for-granted ways of going about one's work may be disrupted by large or small changes. Such changes may result in a quest for order through the construction of checklists and holding a meeting. But when holding a meeting, new suggestions may arise, renewing some sense of disorder, so that another document to bring order can be demanded. This document may quickly be found to be insufficient or in need of revision or interpretation, creating a demand for yet another meeting, and so on, as the administrative spiral continues to perpetuate itself.

New types of rehabilitative ideals, practices, laws, and policies can be seen as efforts to bring order and transparency into human services. In our studies, we have seen that incident reports (aimed to answer "what went wrong?") filed in, for instance, elder care or the social services, create a chain of meeting and document activities to establish when, by whom, and how these reports should be written. Furthermore, a rather straightforward demand for the human services to formulate a so-called Coordinated Individual Plan (SIP), to avoid problems with clients moving around among many agencies, similarly produced a multitude of paperwork in the form of courses, brochures, and papers, on top of (and within) many meetings. Many documents are followed by the production of meta-documentation—documents about the documentation. Similarly, meetings about upcoming or past meetings, and meetings agendas referring to other meetings, can be defined as promising to the pursuit for order and transparency.

Administrative attractions

Designing documents may also harbor intrinsic attractions. Being skillful in producing flowcharts, or diagrams and graphs for that matter, seems to be appreciated and highly valued by professionals. It can be noted in *en passant* comments like, "Wow! You're a pro!" when someone presents their efforts at a meeting in a convincing performance. The professionals we encountered could use one of the numerous software programs that offer tools for creating administrative artwork that looks "professional." "Draw beautiful flowcharts easily and quickly with an online flowchart software," says one of them, thereby implying both the aesthetically appealing and the efficiently professional.

In spite of widespread mutterings about meetings as time-consuming and boring, people often come alive and appear engaged during meetings, even if they sighed before entering them. When "participating" in a meeting without actively engaging, attendees can use their boredom as a background to form alliances and share ironic glances with each other, engage in sneaky work, or find time for side-involvements.

In this concluding discussion, we want to end with some reflections divided into three themes: 1) integrated top-down and bottom-up social forces, 2) a grumbling yet enthusiastic stance, and 3) a Simmelean interactionist approach to capture the hidden attractions of administration.

Top-down and bottom-up

First, we want to acknowledge that even though we have devoted this book to the self-propelling process and inner dynamics that enforce the expanding administration society, these are obviously integrated with the top-down social forces that most researchers mention.

Some of these social scientists explicitly or implicitly criticize the controlling top-down mechanisms such as New Public Management, Audit Society, or the evidence movement. But they do so while succumbing to an idea of cause and effect, in line with, as Nedelmann says (1990:245) "… an age in which everything appears to be able to be controlled and regulated." Rather, she continues, there is a "ceaseless mutual interaction" between cause and effect. Nedelmann's stance, derived from Simmel, is our angle: cause and effect might reverse roles and become embedded in each other, and through such an analytical lens, we may open up new interpretations and a sharpened empirical attentiveness. The processes of social action typical of the modern administration society are tricky, messy, and intrinsically entangled and need more surprising and less taken-for-granted frames or concepts than the linear cause-and-effect logic gives us. Top-down social forces are in play, yes—but inside the organizations and their mundane life, there are more things going on.

Consider, for instance, the myriad regulations that the Swedish National Board for Health and Welfare demands by requiring that all regional and city councils have a "quality steering system." This system applies to all public health and dental care as well as social welfare, as evaluations and control have become increasingly important (SOSFS 2011:9).[2] Consequently, most contemporary social welfare offices nowadays have a wealth of "management bureaucrats" (Hall 2012). Hjärpe (2020:165) illustrates this tendency in an ethnographic study of measurements in social work by relating how she encountered many social workers who had changed their occupation to become quality developers, strategists, planning secretaries, method developers, etc., while still working for the same employer. These are people who now work with writing reports and participating in meetings with other professionals, and who are no longer interacting with clients. In sum: the demand from "the top" for a "quality steering system" is responded to by new professional titles being developed and filled by engaged and motivated people who willingly take on and expand their given administrative tasks. These same people can be expected to further expand these tasks by proposing new methods and policies, thus producing more paperwork and more meetings, and probably also new administrative titles.

Or take the self-propelling mechanism of the Coordinated Care Plans (SIPs), discussed in Chapters 5 and 6, that are now required to be written for those in care to improve collaboration among many agencies. The idea is fairly simple: what needs to be done and who is responsible should be stated for each client in a care plan. There is thus a top-down legal regulation. But instead of merely leading to the formulation of a standard document for each client, this regulation has produced a tremendous amount of meetings, courses, and production of documents initiated from employers and local managers, fueled from below by administrators and staff who will be responsible for the care plan and the meetings that go with it.

Sometimes a new policy from the central level in an organization has to be interpreted and concretized at lower levels, which may result in a chain of meetings. The guidelines must be interpreted. Our interviewees explain that the way they go about it is to arrange meetings, create work-groups, and committees, and produce new local guidelines.

It is obvious that holding a meeting to interpret policies seems to be a contemporary self-evident way of going about decision making. Going back in time, one may imagine an organization that had fewer meetings, that might have been more hierarchical, where a manager decided how the new policy was to be interpreted and organized according to this decision. But as we have noted, meetingization is driven by the trend of involving more employees as part of a process of democratization in contemporary societies.

Representatives of different organizations may also find some attractions in managing top-down documentary demands in creative ways. One such example was given in Chapter 9, *Muddy transparency*, where staff used the incident reports for completely different purposes than intended. Instead of limiting the incident report to things that go wrong, such as deviation from routines that could harm the patient or client, all social workers from a unit agreed to file reports en masse to demonstrate to their superiors what they believed was a far too heavy workload. This action was a result of meetings and materialized in expanding documentation practice.

Other top-down social forces can be found in various management trends launched from above, which may also encourage administrative work from below. One such trend—"Lean"—is mostly associated with staff efficiency.

As noted, this management model has been imported from the car industry into various public organizations, such as hospitals (Radnor et al. 2012). Instead of processing cars efficiently, however, in hospitals, the aim with Lean was to process patients in a well-ordered systematic way (cf. Hedlund forthcoming). How this model has been incorporated into organizations has been studied by Thedvall (2019) in relation to preschools and by Hjärpe (2020) in relation to social work involving child welfare and assistance assessment for the elderly, sick, or disabled. As documented by both Thedvall and Hjärpe, the initiatives to start up Lean came from below, from unit managers. The model was meant to save time but ended up generating more meetings. The new type of Lean meeting was added to the old meetings.

Not only various management models but the human services' rehabilitation models that come and go, can be expected to form the same administrative spiraling processes. Staff have to attend courses, participate in meetings, read and produce programs, documenting rehabilitative progress or lack of progress in relation to treatment programs such as for example "cognitive self-change" (Fox 1999), "tough love" (Lee Burns and Peyrot 2003), or "family work" (Åkerström 2006).

A grumbling yet enthusiastic stance

A second theme we want to reflect on is the contrast between the grumbling about meetings and documents in contrast to the engagement and involvement in such bureaucratic or administrative work. In Chapter 3, *Seductive gatherings*, we described how Nellie, who meets a colleague, sighs, and rolls her eyes when explaining she is on her way to "one of those monthly meetings." But later on, when the meeting has started, Nellie turns out to be one of the most engaged participants.

Even among top managers whose job tasks typically involve meetings and paperwork, such complaints also seem to be common (Bargiela and Harris 1997; Mangset 2019). In one of our studies, of a collaboration among border police organizations financed by the EU (Yakhlef 2020), this tendency was particularly obvious. The many bureaucratic demands conflicted with the ideal image of the police, whose occupational identities celebrate "action" and can be described as pragmatic and demonstratively anti-theoretical (Chan 2004; Loftus 2010; Sausdal forthcoming). Even top managers within police organizations emphasize their "street smartness," "toughness," or past crime-fighting successes, rather than their administrative skills, wisdom as "people managers," or their educational achievements (Manning 2007:70). This also was true for the top managers we followed, but we did see them "coming alive" during the many formal meetings attached to the project, and they often emphasized the importance of various documents in negotiations with each other.

The contrast between sighing over meetings and documents but then engaging in them is not to be taken at face value.[3] In fact, noting this contrast, discovering enthusiasm while reflecting on the common grumblings about bureaucracy and administration, initiated the research that resulted in this book. Inside the contrast there are dynamics that explain the paradox. Such dynamics have been identified and analyzed throughout the book, and include the movement between formality and informality, as well as the movement between involvement and disinvolvement, between control and escape-the-control.

Capturing the hidden attractions of administration

A third theme we want to highlight is more theoretical. Simmel, as Nedelmann pointed out, was interested in the *Eigendynamik* or self-propelling processes as pertaining to a social phenomenon like fashion, where innovation is followed by imitation, creating renewed efforts of innovation, and so on. To attend to *Eigendynamik* is a way to discern social processes that repeat themselves when swinging between poles or contrasts, and according to Nedelmann (1990:245, 253), such processes especially thrive in social phenomena characterized by ambivalence. People feel both attraction and repulsion to fashion, and we find the equivalent emotions in relation to administration. We find it in the interactions in meetings with their particular combination of formalities and informalities, dullness and drama. Local cultures supply accountable behavioral codes for their members to alternate between layers of constraint and liberation, so that an interest in what is happening—"the action" in Goffman's terms (1967/1982:149–270)—can be continually sustained.

The major eigendynamic process we have discussed in this book concerns a pendulum movement that exists between order and disorder. This is the process that leads to a self-generating spiral. We find a range of practices aiming at once-and-for-all ordering of people-processing organizations, only to re-create conditions and situations with a relative sense of disorder that consequently "needs" to be ordered, again.

Meetings generate new meetings because the last one did not seem to cover it all, and in the interaction between meetings and documents, they generate one another. People want to have structure, but also break away from the structures, so they add things on their own and detect things that are not completely covered, thus setting the scene for upcoming efforts to try to make order anew. In Schwartzman's alternative health care organization, where all participants had their say, we see a clear example of a series of endless meetings, propelled by employees yearning for *some* structure. And structure can be promised with the help of documents—which, in turn, eventually are found to be too one-dimensional, rigid, and imprisoning, so that they have to be revised and elaborated. This step in turn may very well make them too expansive, so that we have to specify them again and discuss this in a meeting.

Simmel, whose perspective has inspired this book, is an interactionist, but his emphasis is social phenomena in general, not face-to-face encounters.

We certainly ground a lot of our investigations in narrated and observed face-to-face encounters by using Simmel's observations, as have others (e.g., Bergmann 1993; George 1993; Sellerberg 1994; Tavory 2009), but we also discern interactions in more durable, far-reaching, and encompassing ways, and at a larger scale. People may be enthusiastic about the aesthetics of documents, and they can come alive during a meeting, enjoying the small drama or the joking relations with colleagues that are inserted into the stiff, formal event. But the administration society of today is also driven by other types of interactions: between meetings and documents through emails, invitations, and collective summons; between administrators and other employees through instructions and their teaching ambitions; and between organizations and divisions of organizations.

As we see it, an interactionist perspective is needed to capture today's *Eigendynamik* of administration. It must, however, be Simmelean inter-actionism coupled with empirically detailed observations allowed by Simmel's generosity of forms and scales.

In this book, we have attempted to illustrate the ambivalence that creates Simmel's *Eigendynamik* or autonomous processes between order and dis-order in relation to administration. Today we want schedules, but we also want freedom and improvisation; we want written, structured agendas, but we also want individual expressions and original ideas. We are attracted to both poles, but we also reject them, so that when one is reached, we become a bit dissatisfied and start striving for the other. This is how the adminis-trative spiral self-generates its power. And this is how the client in human services organizations is put in the shadow, whereas the palace of admin-istration gets shinier and shinier.

Notes

1 Lacking documents can also open the "wrong door." The consequences of lacking the magic brought about by signing the correct document might land you in some difficulties, which was the case for a Chinese tourist who lost his wallet in Germany. When he signed the wrong paperwork, he ended up being placed in a refugee home. "It took German officials 12 days to put the story together and send the 31-year-old tourist on his way." https://apnews.com/article/9857d1d27320448b93eeb233a3a8d9c1 [Retrieved 2020-02-07]

2 SOSFS 2011:9. Ledningssystem för systematiskt kvalitetsarbete. [Management system for systematic quality work]. The Swedish National Board for Health and Welfare. https://www.socialstyrelsen.se/globalassets/sharepoint-dokument/artikelkatalog/foreskrifter-och-allmanna-rad/2011-6-38.pdf [Retrieved 2020-09-29]

3 Rogelberg, Scott, and Kello (2007) have noted this disparity in a quantitative study. People often complained about meetings, but when asked about the "productivity" of their last meeting a majority rated them positively. These authors do not, however, try to explain the dynamics of these occasions.

Appendix: Methods and materials

Inspired by Simmel's formal sociology and Vaughan's (2004, 2015) Simmel-informed analytical ethnography, we have extracted analytical and theoretical traces from different ethnographic case studies through analogical theorizing. This means that we strive to compare activities, phenomena, or experiences of different empirical fields, which may harbor similar sociological traits. Both qualitative similarities and differences in our social phenomenon—hidden attractions of administration—have been included when generalizing findings from different empirical fields: health care, the social services, public youth care, psychiatric care, and border police cooperation. Most of our material are generated and collected from human services organizations, but we have also interviewed heads of university departments and taken fieldnotes from our own habitat, academia, while working with this book.

All of our case studies are conducted ethnographically with participant observation as the main method; we have shadowed professionals during workdays (Czarniawska 2007), conducted "go-alongs" (Kusenbach 2003) with managers to attend meetings at other agencies, and "sit-alongs" by the computer asking the professionals to think aloud while filling out forms for example. This material is supplemented with interviews, mostly with professionals: doctors, nurses, social workers, detention home teachers, to mention but a few, some of them in the capacity as quality coordinators and managers. To a lesser extent the material consists of interviews with clients, namely young people in care and drug addicts. Interviews were recorded and carried out in a conversational style. They are transcribed verbatim, and the quotations used in this article were translated into English in a way that preserves the original meaning and style. Thus, the translation is not literal, and the word order has been altered to follow Standard English usage. Departing from an ethnographic approach to documents and an interest in documents-in-use (Jacobsson forthcoming), we have collected documents that were important to members in different field sites and often routinely used.

The analyses carried out for this book are based on empirical material from a number of studies that we have already reported, but for the purpose of this book we now "recycled" the same data with new questions in mind (Wästerfors, Åkerström, and Jacobsson 2014). Material from some case

DOI: 10.4324/9781003108436-102

studies are more quoted than others, but all cases have been influential for the ideas underpinning this book. In addition, we have collected and generated new material specifically for this book project. In summary, the book is based on the following case studies carried out by the authors and collaborators.

Case study 1: investigation of a project in youth care

The study consisted of a collaborative project between SiS youth care and the municipalities' social services, directed by The National Board of Institutional Care. During the project, extensive empirical material was collected in the form of interviews (a total of 145) with parents, young people, coordinators, department staff, and employees in social administrations. In addition, 70 days of shadowing the coordinators' workdays as well as observation of meetings and go-alongs are included (Basic, Thelander, and Åkerström 2009; Thelander and Åkerström 2019; Åkerström 2017, 2019; Åkerström and Wästerfors forthcoming).

Case study 2: a study of border police meetings

The study examines a two-year-long collaborative project between the border police in Estonia, Finland, Latvia, Lithuania, and Sweden. This included a longer fieldwork (approximately 700 hours of field observations) and a large number of interviews, just over 70 (Yakhlef 2020; Åkerström, Wästerfors, and Yakhlef 2020).

Case study 3: paperwork in primary care and the social services

In a four-year-long project on documentary realities we shadowed workers in three primary care centers and three social service units, as well as interviewed professionals and clients. We also followed a one-year leadership course for managers in the social services. Documents used by the participants were collected extensively (Jacobsson and Martinell Barfoed 2019; Jacobsson and Thelander 2016; Hjärpe 2019, 2020; Carlstedt and Jacobsson 2017; Martinell Barfoed 2019; Jacobsson 2016).

Case study 4: meeting activities in psychiatry

In a joint project on meetings, both interviews and field observations were carried out in the form of go-alongs with managers in a psychiatric clinic (Leppänen 2018; Thelander 2017; Thelander and Åkerström 2019).

Case study 5: school work at detention homes

This project gathered almost a hundred qualitative interviews with pedagogical leaders, pupils, and teachers at five detention homes in Sweden, in addition to extensive fieldnotes from participant observations of classroom teaching and surrounding situations. Most interviews were conducted face-to-face, but 21 pedagogical leaders at different institutions all over Sweden were interviewed over the phone (Wästerfors 2014, 2018).

Case study 6: observations of social worker-client assessment interviews

In this study, we collected various data concerning the standardized assessment of social service needs in eight cases: individual interviews with the social worker and the client, audio recordings of the assessment interview with the client carried out by the social worker, follow-up interviews when the results from the standardized interview was interpreted by the social worker. In addition, three days in-service training for social workers was followed (e.g., Martinell Barfoed and Jacobsson 2012; Martinell Barfoed 2018).

Case study 7: decision-making at a cardiology clinic

This study generated two months of observations at a cardiology clinic along with eight recorded interviews with the nurses and doctors shadowed, to enable more time for undisturbed talk about what had happened during the observations. Staff meetings, morning rounds, and handover meetings involved a large amount of documents utilized by the staff in various ways (Avendal and Jacobsson 2012; Jacobsson 2013, 2014).

Case study 8: violence in detention homes

This study builds on qualitative interviews with staff and young people on their experiences of violent events, and how to manage and avoid them. Around 15 events were studied up close, including interviews with the involved young people and staff members. In addition, journal notes and incident reports were collected, and new as well as previously collected fieldnotes were used. Moreover, 27 other inmates and staff members were interviewed on conflicts in general (14 young people and 13 staff members). In total, the study includes at least 71 interviews from seven detention homes (Wästerfors 2019a, 2019b).

Case study 9: managing conflicts in detention homes

This study consists of ethnographic fieldnotes from repeated visits at one detention home, including everyday life, small talk, and field-based interviews. In addition, 20 qualitative interviews were conducted (including 12 staff members and 11 young people) and journal notes about 11 young people in care were collected (Wästerfors and Åkerström 2015; Wästerfors 2009, 2011, 2012, 2014).

Case study 10: academic managers on meetings

Conversational interviews were carried out with academic managers from various departments and administrations at both universities and colleges. A total of nine heads of university and college institutions and administrations have been interviewed about how they view meetings and their memories of them (Andersson Cederholm and Åkerström 2020; Thelander and Åkerström 2019).

Case study 11: observations at a substance abuse treatment center

Participant observation and collection of documents at a substance abuse treatment center. The researcher attended all meetings of various kinds during a week to participate in the center's everyday meeting rhythm.

Case study 12: managers in The National Board of Institutional Care

The survey included ten days of field observations when managers at The National Board of Institutional Care's youth institutions were "shadowed" during their work days, and we collected their calendars. In addition, five of these were interviewed.

References

Abram, Simone (2017). Contradictions in contemporary political life: Meeting bureaucracy in Norwegian municipal government. Pp. 27–44 in *Meetings: Ethnographies of Organizational Process, Bureaucracy, and Assembly*. Hanna Brown, Adam Reed, and Thomas Yarrow (Eds.). Journal of the Royal Anthropological Institute, Special Issue Book Series. Hoboken, NJ: Wiley-Blackwell.

Abram, Simone (2017). Learning to meet (or how to talk to chairs). Pp. 63–90 in *Meeting Ethnography. Meetings as Key Technologies of Contemporary Governance, Development, and Resistance*. Jen Sandler and Renita Thedvall (Eds.). New York: Routledge.

Abramovitz, Mimi (2005). The largely untold story of welfare reform and the human services. *Social Work*, 50(2): 175–186.

Agevall, Ola and Gunnar Olofsson (2020). Administratörerna: Administration, kontroll och styrning vid svenska universitet och högskolor. *Arkiv*, 12: 7–59.

Ahmed, Sara (2007). "You end up doing the document rather than doing the doing": Diversity, race equality and the politics of documentation. *Ethnic and Racial Studies*, 30(4): 590–609.

Akerström, Malin (2006). Doing ambivalence: Embracing policy innovation—at arm's length. *Social Problems*, 53(1): 57–74.

Akerström, Malin (2017). Mötesstrider och dokumentkamp i ungdomsvården. Pp. 233–257 in *Den motspänstiga akademikern*. Björn Andersson, Frida Petersson and Anette Skårner (Eds.). Malmö: Egalité.

Akerström, Malin (2019). The merry–go–round of meetings: Embracing meetings in a Swedish youth care project. *Sociological Focus*, 52(1): 50–64.

Akerström, Malin and David Wästerfors (forthcoming). Ethnographic discovery after fieldwork. In *Doing Human Service Ethnography*. Jaber F. Gubrium and Katarina Jacobsson (Eds.). Bristol, UK: Policy Press.

Akerström, Malin and Katarina Jacobsson (Eds.) (2019). "Producing people" in documents and meetings in human service organizations. *Social Inclusion*, 7(1):180–184.

Akerström, Malin; David Wästerfors, and Sophia Yakhlef (2020). Meetings or power weeks? Boundary work in a transnational police project. *Qualitative Sociology Review*, 16(3): 70–84.

Allen, Davina (2000). Doing occupational demarcation: The "boundary-work" of nurse managers in a district general hospital. *Journal of Contemporary Ethnography*, 29(3): 326–356.

Allen, Joseph A; Nale Lehmann-Willenbrock, and Steven G. Rogelberg (Eds.) (2015). *The Cambridge Handbook of Meeting Science*. New York: Cambridge University Press.

DOI: 10.4324/9781003108436-103

Alvesson, Mats (2019). *Extra allt!: när samhälls- och människoförbättrandet slår tillbaka.* Stockholm: Fri tanke.

Anderson, Gina (2006). Carving out time and space in the managerial university. *Journal of Organizational Change Management*, 19(4): 578–592.

Andersson Cederholm, Erika (2010). Effective emotions–the enactment of a work ethic in the Swedish meeting industry. *Culture Unbound: Journal of Current Cultural Research*, 2(3): 381–400.

Andersson Cederholm, Erika and Patrik Hall (2020). Performing ambiguous policy: How innovation events simultaneously perform change and collaborative order. *The Sociological Review*, 68(6): 1403–1419.

Andersson Cederholm, Erika and Malin Åkerström (2020). Calender elicitation–uncovering the taken-for-granted routines of workplace meetings. Unsubmitted manuscript.

Askeland, Gurid Aga and Helle Strauss (2014). The Nordic welfare model, civil society and social work. Pp. 241–254 in *Global Social Work: Crossing Borders, Blurring Boundaries*. Noble Carolyn, Strauss Helle and Littlechild Brian (Eds.). Sydney: Sydney University Press.

Asmuß, Birte and Jan Svennevig (2009). Meeting talk: An introduction. *The Journal of Business Communication*, 46(1): 3–22.

Atkinson, Mick A; Edward C. Cuff, and John R. E. Lee (1978). The recommencement of a meeting as a member's accomplishment. Pp. 133–153 in *Studies in the Organization of Conversational Interaction*. Jim Schenken (Ed.) New York: Academic Press.

Avendal, Christel and Katarina Jacobsson (2012). *Beslutsfattande i sjukvården–en forskningsöversikt*. Research Reports in Social Work, 2012:1. School of Social Work, Lund University.

Bachrach, Peter and S. Baratz Morton (1963). Decisions and nondecisions: An analytical framework. *American Political Science Review*, 57(3): 632–642.

Baines, Donna (2006). Whose needs are being served? Quantitative metrics and the re-shaping of social services. *Studies in Political Economy*, 77(1): 95–209.

Barbalet, Jack M (1999). Boredom and social meaning. *British Journal of Sociology*, 50(4): 631–646.

Barnets och ungdomens reform (2017). Slutrapport från den nationella samordnaren för den sociala barn- och ungdomsvården. Regeringskansliet: Socialdepartementet. https://www.regeringen.se/4b007c/contentassets/37d51abb4e8c40928c289f4c3b423c37/barnet-och-ungdomens-reform--forslag-for-en-hallbar-framtid.pdf. Retrieved 2021-02-05.

Bargiela, Francesca and Sandra J. Harris (1997). *Managing language: The discourse of corporate meetings*. Philadelphia: John Benjamins.

Basic, Goran (2018). Observed successful collaboration in social work practice: Coherent triads in Swedish juvenile care. *European Journal of Social Work*, 21(2): 193–206.

Basic, Goran; Joakim Thelander, and Malin Åkerström (2009). *Vårdkedja för ungdomar eller professionella?* Stockholm: Statens institutionsstyrelse.

Berger, Peter and Thomas Luckman (1991). *The social construction of reality*. London: Penguin Books.

Bergmann, Jörg (1993). *Discreet indiscretions: The social organization of gossip*. New Brunswick, NJ: Transaction Pub.

Best, Joel (2006). *Flavor of the month*. Berkeley, CA: University of California Press.

Best, Joel (2012). *Damned lies and statistics. Untangling numbers from the media, politicians, and activists*. Berkeley, CA: University of California Press.

Blomgren, Maria (2007). The drive for transparency: Organizational field transformation in Swedish Healthcare. *Public Administration*, 85(1): 67–82.

Boden, Deidre (1994). *The business of talk: Organizations in action.* Cambridge: Polity.

Bohlin, Ingemar and Morten Sager (2011). *Evidensens många ansikten.* Lund: Arkiv.

Bowker, Geoffrey C. and Susan Leigh Star (1999). *Sorting things out. Classification and its consequences.* Cambridge, MA: The MIT Press.

Brodkin, Evelyn and Malay Majumdar (2010). Administrative exclusion: Organizations and the hidden costs of welfare claiming. *Journal of Public Administration Research and Theory,* 20: 827–848.

Bromley, Patricia and John Meyer (2015). *Hyper-Organizations–Global organizational expansion.* Oxford: Oxford University Press.

Brown, Hanna; Adam Reed, and Thomas Yarrow (Eds.) (2017). *Meetings: Ethnographies of organizational process, bureaucracy, and assembly.* Journal of the Royal Anthropological Institute, Special Issue Book Series. Hoboken, NJ: Wiley-Blackwell.

Bruno, Isabelle; Emmanuel Didier, and Tommaso Vitale (2014). Statactivism: Forms of action between disclosure and affirmation. *The Open Journal of Sociopolitical Studies,* 7(2): 198–220.

Brunsson, Nils (2006). *Mechanisms of hope: Maintaining the dream of the rational organization.* Malmö: Liber.

Burns, Stacy Lee and Mark Peyrot (2003). Tough love: Nurturing and coercing responsibility and recovery in California drug courts. *Social Problems,* 50(3): 416–438.

Bäsén, Anna (2003). *Vem ska ta hand om min mamma? Min dagbok inifrån äldrevården.* Stockholm: Bokförlaget Forum.

Carlstedt, Elisabeth and Katarina Jacobsson (2017). Indications of quality or quality as a matter of fact? "Open Comparisons" within the social work sector. *Statsvetenskaplig Tidskrift,* 2017(1): 47–69.

Cross, Rob; Reb Rebele and Adam Grant (2016). Collaborative Overload. *Harvard Business Review,* (January–February): 74–79. https://hbr.org/2016/01/collaborative-overload.

Czarniawska, Barbara (2007). *Shadowing: And other techniques for doing fieldwork in modern societies.* Copenhagen: Copenhagen Business School Press.

Czarniawska-Joerges, Barbara (1992). *Exploring complex organizations: A cultural perspective.* Newbury Park, CA: Sage Publications.

Darden, Donna and Alan Marks (1999). Boredom: A socially disvalued emotion. *Sociological Spectrum,* 19(1): 13–37.

The Economist (2018). "The rise of universities' diversity bureaucrats" *The Economist* explains. Retrieved 2018-05-08. https://www.economist.com/the-economist-explains/2018/05/08/the-rise-of-universities-diversity-bureaucrats.

Eggen, Oyvind (2012). Performing Good Governance: The aesthetics of bureaucratic practice in Malawi. *Ethnos,* 77(1): 1–23.

Enell, Sofia; Sabine Gruber, and Maria Andersson Vogel (2018). *Kontrollerade unga: tvångspraktiker på institution.* Lund: Studentlitteratur.

Erickson, Shari; Brooke Rockwern, Michelle Koltov, and Robert M. McLean (2017). Putting patients first by reducing administrative tasks in health care. *Annals of Internal Medicine,* 166(9): 659–661.

Eriksson-Zetterquist, Ulla; Alexander Styhre, and Thomas Kalling (2015). *Organisation och organisering.* Malmö: Liber.

Espeland, Wendy N. and Mitchell L. Stevens (2008). A sociology of quantification. *European Journal of Sociology,* 49(3): 401–436.

Fairclough, Norman (1993). Critical discourse analysis and the marketization of public discourse: The Universities. *Discourse and Society,* 4(2): 133–168.

Farrell, Catherine and Jonathan Morris (1999). Markets, bureaucracy and public management: Professional perceptions of bureaucratic change in the public sector: GPs, headteachers and social workers. *Public Money and Management*, 19(4): 31–36.

Fine, Gary Alan and Ugo Corte (2017). Group pleasures: Collaborative commitments, shared narrative, and the sociology of fun. *Sociological Theory*, 35(1): 64–86.

Flaherty, Michael (2011). *The textures of time. Agency and temporal experience.* Philadelphia, PA: Temple University Press.

Flower, Lisa (2019). *Interactional justice: The role of emotions in the performance of loyalty.* London: Routledge.

Flyverbom, Mikkel (2016). Transparency: Mediation and the Management of Visibilities. *International Journal of Communication*, 10: 110–122.

Forssell, Anders and Anders Ivarsson Westerberg (2014). *Administrationssamhället.* Lund: Studentlitteratur.

Fox, Kathryn (1999). Changing violent minds: Discursive correction and resistance in the cognitive treatment of violent offenders in prison. *Social Problems*, 46(1): 88–103.

Garsten, Christina and Kerstin Jacobsson (2016). Transparency as ideal and practice: Labour market policy and audit culture in the Swedish public employment service. *Statsvetenskaplig tidskrift*, 118(1): 69–92.

George, Kenneth (1993). Dark trembling: Ethnographic notes on secrecy and concealment in highland Sulawesi. *Anthropological Quarterly*, 66(4): 230–239.

Goffman, Erving (1959). *The presentation of self in everyday life.* Garden City, NY: Anchor.

Goffman, Erving (1967/1982). *Interaction ritual.* Chicago: Aldine.

Goffman, Erving (1974). *Frame analysis: An essay on the organization of experience.* New York: Harper and Row.

Goldman, Laurie and Erica Foldy (2015). The space before action. *Social Service Review*, 89: 166–202.

Gubrium, Jaber F. and James A. Holstein (2009). *Analyzing narrative reality.* London: Sage.

Göpfert, Mirco (2013). Bureaucratic aesthetics: Report writing in the Nigérian gendarmerie. *American Ethnologist*, 40(2): 324–334.

Hall, Chris; Stef Slembrouck, and Srikanth Sarangi (2006). *Language practices in social work.* New York: Routledge.

Hall, Patrik (2012). *Managementbyråkrati: Organisationspolitisk makt i svensk offentlig förvaltning.* Malmö: Liber.

Hall, Patrik (2020). Tillväxten av managementbyråkrati–ett hot mot välfärdsstaten? Pp. 171–194 in *Statlig förvaltningspolitik för 2020-talet.* Malmö: Statskontoret.

Hall, Patrik; Vesa Leppänen, and Malin Åkerström (2019). *Mötesboken–analyser av arbetslivets sammanträden och rosévinsmingel.* [The Book on Meeting – Analyses of working life's solemn meetings and rose wine mingling] Malmö: Egalité.

Hedlund, David (forthcoming). *The secrets of success. An explorative case-study on how Lean makes magic in Swedish eldercare.* Doctoral Dissertation, School of Social work, Lund University.

Herzfeld, Michael (1992). *The social production of indifference: Exploring the symbolic roots of western bureaucracy.* Chicago: University of Chicago Press.

Hjärpe, Teres (2019). Social work on the whiteboard: Governing by comparing performance. *Social Inclusion*, 7(1): 185–195.

Hjärpe, Teres (2020). *Mätning och motstånd: Sifferstyrning i socialtjänstens vardag.* [Measurement and resistance–Governing social workers by numbers]. Doctoral Dissertation, School of Social Work, Lund University. http://lup.lub.lu.se/record/40a723ea-da90-4435-ab45-e373d0b12c9a.

Hodgson, Damian; Mats Fred, Simon Bailey, and Patrik Hall (Eds.) (2019). *The projectification of the public sector.* London: Routledge.

Hoe, Siu Loon (2019). The topicality of the learning organization: Is the concept still relevant today? Pp. 1–22 in *The Oxford Handbook of the Learning Organization.* Anders Ragnar Örtenblad (Ed.). Oxford: Oxford University Press.

Höglund, Anna and Bengt-Åke Armelius (2003). *Psykosocial arbetsmiljö hos administrativ personal.* [The psychosocial work environment among adminstrative staff]. Research report. Department of Psychology, Umeå University, 2003:3.

Hood, Christopher (1991). A public management for all seasons? *Public Administration,* 69(1): 3–19.

Hood, Christopher and Ruth Dixon (2015). What we have to show for 30 years of new public management: Higher costs, more complaints. *Governance,* 28(3): 265–267.

Hughes, Everett C (1963). Professions. *Daedalus,* 92(4): 655–668.

Hughes, Everett C (1984). *The sociological eye.* New Brunswick, NJ: Transaction Books.

Høybye-Mortensen, Matilde, (2015). Social work and artefacts: Social workers' use of objects in client relations. European Journal of Social Work, 18(5): 703–717. Hughes, Everett C (1963). Professions. *Daedalus,* 92(4): 655–668.

Ivarsson Westerberg, Anders (2004). *Papperspolisen: Den ökande administrationen i moderna organisationer.* Doctoral Dissertation. Handelshögskolan, Stockholm. urn:nbn:se:sh: diva-9034

Ivarsson Westerberg, Anders and Bengt Jacobsson (2013). *Staten och granskningssamhället.* Stockholm: Förvaltningsakademin.

Jacobsson, Katarina (2013). En förtjänt patient? Moraliska bedömningar i sjukvården. *Socialmedicinsk tidskrift,* 90(1): 179–188.

Jacobsson, Katarina (2014). Categories by heart: Shortcut reasoning in a cardiology clinic. *Professions and Professionalism,* 4(3): 1–15.

Jacobsson, Katarina (2016). Analysing documents through fieldwork. Pp. 155–170 in *Qualitative research* (4th ed.). David Silverman (Ed.). London: Sage.

Jacobsson, Katarina and Elizabeth Martinell Barfoed (2019). *Socialt arbete och pappersgöra.* [Social work and paperwork]. Malmö: Gleerups.

Jacobsson, Katarina and Anna Meeuwisse (2020). "State governing of knowledge"–Constraining social work research and practice. *European Journal of Social Work,* 23(2): 277–289.

Jacobsson, Katarina and Joakim Thelander (2016). *Den motvillige administratören. Om datorjobb och pappersgöra på vårdcentralen.* Research Reports in Social Work, 2016: 3, Socialhögskolan: Lunds universitet, Lund.

Jacobsson, Kerstin (2004). Soft regulation and the subtle transformation of states: the case of EU employment policy. *Journal of European Social Policy,* 14(4): 355–370.

Katz, Jack (1990). *Seductions of Crime: Moral and Sensual Attractions in Doing Evil.* New York: Basic Books.

Katz, Jack (1999). *How Emotions Work.* Chicago: Chicago University Press.

Kello, John (2015). The science and practice of workplace meetings. Pp. 709–734 in *The Cambridge Handbook of Meeting Science.* A. Joseph, Allen Nale Lehmann-Willenbrock and Steven G. Rogelberg (Eds.). New York: Cambridge University Press.

Kjellberg, Inger (2019). Klagomålsfunktionen. Pp. 103–117 in *Perspektiv på granskning inom offentlig sektor.* Anders Hanberger och Lena Lindgren (Eds.). Malmö: Gleerups.

Kleinman, Lisa (2010). *Physically present, mentally absent? Technology multitasking in organizational meetings.* Doctoral Dissertation. The University of Texas, Austin. https:// repositories.lib.utexas.edu/handle/2152/ETD-UT-2010-05-800.

Kunda, Gideon (2006). *Engineering Culture*. Philadelphia, PA: Temple University.

Kusenbach, Margarethe (2003). Street phenomenology: The go–along as ethnographic research tool. *Ethnography*, 4(3): 455–485.

Lamont, Michéle and Viràg Molnár (2002). The study of boundaries in the social sciences. *Annual Review of Sociology*, 28(1): 167–195.

Lamp, Nicolas (2017). The receding horizon of informality in WTO meetings. *Journal of Royal Anthropological Institute*, 23(S1): 63–79.

Lascoumes, Pierre and Patrick Le Gales (2007). Introduction: Understanding public policy through its instruments. *Governance*, 20(1): 1–21.

Lauri, Marcus (2016). *Narratives of governing: Rationalization, responsibility and resistance in social work*. Doctoral Dissertation. Department of Political Science and Umeå Centre for Gender Studies, Umeå University. urn:nbn:se:umu:diva-119783.

Lindgren, Lena (2014). *Nya utvärderingsmonstret: Om kvalitetsmätning i den offentliga sektorn*. [The new evaluation monster: On measuring quality in the public sector]. Lund: Studentlitteratur.

Lindgren, Torgny (1973). *Övriga frågor*. Stockholm: Norstedts.

Lipsky, Michael (1980). *Street-level bureaucracy*. New York: Russell Sage Foundation.

Ljung, Mikael and Anders Ivarsson Westerberg (2017). *När målstyrning blev detaljstyrning: Arbetsvillkor och administrativa rutiner i hemtjänsten*. Förvaltningsakademin: Södertörns högskola.

Mangset, Marte and Kristin Asdal (2019). Bureaucratic power in note-writing: Authoritative expertise within the state. *British Journal of Sociology*, 70(2): 569–588.

Manning, Peter (2007). A dialectic of organizational and ocuppational culture. Pp. 47–83 in *Police Occupational Culture*. Megan O'Neill, Monique Marks, and Anne-Marie Sing (Eds.) Amsterdam: Elsevier.

Martinell Barfoed, Elizabeth (2018). From stories to standardised interaction–Changing conversational formats in social work. *Nordic Social Work Research*, 8(1): 36–49.

Martinell Barfoed, Elizabeth (2019). Digital clients: An example of people production in social work. *Social Inclusion*, 7(1): 196–206.

Martinell Barfoed, Elizabeth and Katarina Jacobsson (2012). Moving from "gut feeling" to "pure facts": Launching the ASI interview as part of in-service training for social workers. *Nordic Social Work Research*, 2(1): 5–20.

Mauss, Marcel (2001). *A general theory of magic*. London: Routledge.

Merton, Robert K. (1976). *Sociological ambivalence and other essays*. New York: Free Press.

Nedelmann, Birgitta (1990). Georg Simmel as an analyst of autonomous dynamics. Pp. 243–257 in *George Simmel and Contemporary Sociology*. Bernard Michael Kearn, S. Phillips and S. Cohen Robert (Eds.). London: Kluwer Academic Publishers.

Nordström, Erik (2016). *Samordnad individuell plan (SIP): Professionellas samt barn och föräldrars erfarenheter*. Doctoral thesis. School of Health and Welfare, Jönköping. http://hj.diva-portal.org/smash/record.jsf?pid=diva2%3A951970&dswid=1472.

Olien, Jessie Lynn; Steven G. Rogelberg, Nale Lehmann-Willenbrock, and Joseph A. Allen (2015). Exploring meeting science. Pp. 12–19 in *The Cambridge Handbook of Meeting Science*. Joseph A. Allen, Nale Lehmann-Willenbrock and Steven G. Rogelberg (Eds.). New York: Cambridge University Press.

O'Malley, Pat; Lorna Weir, and Clifford Shearing (1997). Governmentality, criticism, politics. *Economy and Society*, 26(4): 501–517.

Ortenblad, Anders Ragnar (Ed.) (2019). *The Oxford handbook of the learning organization*. Oxford: Oxford University Press.

Peck, Edward; Perri Six, Pauline Gulliver, and David Towell (2004). Why do we keep on meeting like this? The board as ritual in health and social care. *Health Services Management Ressearch*, 17(2): 100–109.

Polletta, Francesca (2002). *Freedom is an endless meeting: Democracy in American social movements*. Chicago: University of Chicago Press.

Power, Michael (1997). *Audit society: Rituals of verification*. Oxford: Oxford University Press.

Prior, Lindsay (2003). *Using documents in social research*. London: Sage.

Radnor, Zoe; Matthias Holweg, and Justin Waring (2012). Lean in healthcare: The unfilled promise? *Social Science & Medicine*, 74(3): 364–371.

Riessman Kohler, Catherine (2002). Analysis of personal narratives. Pp. 695–710 in *Handbook of Interview Research*. Jaber F. Gubrium and James A. Holstein (Eds.). London: Sage.

Riles, Annelise (1998). Infinity within the brackets. *American Ethnologist*, 25(3): 378–398.

Rogelberg, Steven G; Cliff Scott, and John Kello (2007). The science and fiction of meetings. *MIT Sloan Management Review*, 48(2): 18.

Rogerson-Revell, Pamela (2007). Humor in business: A double-edged sword. A study of humor and style shifting in intercultural meetings. *Journal of Pragmatics*, 39: 4–28.

Rönnqvist, Jakob (2019). *Samverkan på pappret. En studie om hur primärvård och socialtjänst samverkar med samordnade individuella planer*. Master thesis. School of Social Work, Lund University.

Safian, Shelly C (2009). *Essentials of healthcare compliance*. New York: Delmar Cengage Learning.

Sandler, Jen (2011). Re–framing the politics of urban feeding in U.S. public schools: Parents, programs, activists, and the state. Pp. 25–45 in *School Food Politics: The Complex Ecology of Hunger and Feeding in Schools Around the World*. Sara A. Robert and Marcus B. Weaver–Hightower (Eds.). New York: Peter Lang.

Sausdal, David (forthcoming). Looking Beyond the Police-as-Control Narrative. In *Doing Human Service Ethnography*. Jaber F. Gubrium and Katarina Jacobsson (Eds.). Bristol, U.K: Policy Press.

Scheler, Max (1992). *On feeling, knowing, and valuing*. H. Bershady (Ed.). Chicago: University of Chicago Press.

Schwartzman, Helen B. (1989). *The meeting*. Boston, MA: Springer.

Schwartzman, Helen B. (2015). There's something about meetings: Order and disorder in the study of meetings. Pp. 735–746 in *The Cambridge Handbook of Meeting Science*. Joseph Allen, Nale Lehmann-Willenbrock and Steven G. Rogelberg (Eds.). New York: Cambridge University Press.

Sellerberg, Ann-Mari (1994). *A blend of contradictions: Georg Simmel in theory and practice*. New Brunswick, NJ: Transaction Pub.

Senge, Peter (1990). *The Fifth Discipline: The art and practice of the learning organization*. New York: Doubleday.

Shore, Chris and Susan Wright (2015). Governing by numbers: Audit culture, rankings and the new world order. *Social Anthropology*, 23(1): 22–28.

Simmel, George (1904/1957). Fashion. *American Journal of Sociology*, 62(6): 541–558.

Simmel, George (1964). *Conflict and the web of group affiliation*. Translated by Kurt Wolff and Reinhard Bendix. New York: The Free Press.

Simmel, George (1978). *The philosophy of money*. London: Routledge.

SOU (2016:89). *För digitalisering i tiden*. [Governmental offical report: Towards the digital society]. Stockholm: Digitaliseringskommissionen.

Strathern, Marilyn (2000). The tyranny of transparency. *British Educational Research Journal*, 26(3): 309–321.

Tavory, Iddo (2009). The structure of flirtation: On the construction of interactional ambiguity. Pp. 59–74 in *Studies in Symbolic Interaction Vol. 33*. Norman K. Denzin (Ed.). Bingley: Emerald Group Publishing.

Taylor, Tiffany (2013). Paperwork first, not work first: How caseworkers use paperwork to feel effective. *Journal of Sociology and Social Welfare*, 40(1): 9–28.

Tepper, Steven J (2004). Setting agendas and designing alternatives: Policymaking and the strategic role of meetings. *Review of Policy Research*, 21(4): 523–542.

Thedvall, Renita (2019). *Fast childcare in public preschools: The utopia of efficiency*. London: Routledge.

Thelander, Joakim and Malin Åkerström (2019). Ruled by the calender? Public sector and university managers on meetings, calenders and time. *Sociologisk forskning*, 56(2): 149–165.

Timmermans, Stefan and Marc Berg (2003). *The gold standard: The challenge of evidence-based medicine*. Philadephia: Temple University Press.

Timmermans, Stefan and Steven Epstein (2010). A world of standards but not a standard world: Towards a sociology of standards and standardization. *Annual Review of Sociology*, 36: 69–89.

Vaughan, Dianne (2004). Theorizing disaster: Analogy, historical ethnography, and the challenger accident. *Ethnography*, 5(3): 313–345.

Vaughan, Dianne (2015). Theorizing: Analogy, cases, and comparative social organization. Pp. 61–84 in *Theorizing in Social Science*. Richard Swedberg (Ed.). Stanford: Stanford University Press.

van Vree, Wilbert (1999). *Meetings, manners, and civilization: The development of modern meeting behaviour*. London: Leicester University Press.

van Vree, Wilbert (2011). Meetings: The frontline of civilization. *Sociological Review*, 59(1): 241–262.

Wasson, Christina (2006). Being in two spaces at once. *Journal of Linguistic Anthropology*, 16(1): 103–130.

Weber, Max (1958). *The Protestant ethic and the spirit of capitalism*. Talcott Parsons (transl.; original work published 1903). New York: Charles Scribner.

Weber, Max (1978). *Economy and society*. Guenther Roth and Claus Wittich (Eds.). Vol. 2. Berkeley, CA: University of California Press.

White, Sue; Chris Hall, and Sue Peckover (2009). The descriptive tyranny of the common assessment framework: Technologies of categorization and professional practice in child welfare. *British Journal of Social Work*, 39(7): 1197–1217.

Widmark, Catharina (2015). *Divergent conceptions: Obstacles to collaboration in addressing the needs of children and adolescents*. Doctoral thesis. Karolinska Institutet. https://openarchive. ki.se/xmlui/handle/10616/44744.

Wolcott, Harry F. (2003). *The man in the principal's office: An ethnography*. Maryland, Lanham: Rowman & Altamira.

Wästerfors, David (2009). *Konflikthantering i ungdomsvård ur ett sociologiskt perspektiv*. Stockholm: Statens institutionsstyrelse.

Wästerfors, David (2011). Disputes and going concerns in an institution for "troublesome" boys. *Journal of Contemporary Ethnography*, 40(1): 39–70.

Wästerfors, David (2012). Analyzing social ties in total institutions. *Qualitative Sociology Review*, 8(2): 11–27.

Wästerfors, David (2014). *Lektioner i motvind. Om skola för unga på institution. Malmö*: Égalité.

Wästerfors, David (2018). Taggtråd, soffa och skola. Kampen om undervisning på särskilda ungdomshem. Pp. 191–212 in *Kontrollerade unga. Tvångspraktiker på institution*. Sofia Enell, Sabine Gruber and Maria A. Vogel (Eds.). Lund: Studentlitteratur.

Wästerfors, David (2019a). Things left unwritten. Interview accounts versus institutional texts in a case of detention home violence. *Social Inclusions*, 7(1): 248–258.

Wästerfors, David (2019b). *Vanskligt och kort. Om våldshändelser bland unga på institution*. Lund: Studentlitteratur.

Wästerfors, David and Malin Åkerström (2016). Case history discourse: A rhetoric of troublesome youngsters and faceless treatment. *European Journal of Social Work*, 19(6): 871–886.

Wästerfors, David; Malin Åkerström, and Katarina Jacobsson (2014). Reanalysis of qualitative data. Pp. 467–480 in *The Sage Handbook of Qualitative Data Analysis*. Uwe Flick (Ed.). London: Sage.

Yakhlef, Sophia (2020). *Cross-border police collaboration – Building communities of practice in the Baltic Sea area*. London: Routledge.

Yoerger, Michael; Francis Kyle, and Joseph Allen (2015). So much more than 'chit-chat' – A closer look at premeeting talk. Pp. 153–173 in *The Cambridge Handbook of Meeting Science*. Joseph Allen, Nale Lehmann-Willenbrock and Steven G. Rogelberg (Eds.). New York: Cambridge University Press.

Index

DOI: 10.4324/9781003108436-104